1 0 0 0
COSORI

AIR FRYER TOASTER
OVEN COMBO

COOKBOOK

1000 DAYS FRESH AND FOOLPROOF RECIPES FOR YOUR
COSORI AIR FRYER TOASTER OVEN COMBO

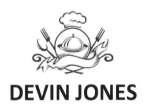

DEVIN JONES

CONTENTS

INTRODUCTION

How Does the COSORI Air Fryer Oven Work?

An air fryer oven takes the latest craze of air fryers that use convection heat to cook rapidly in a confined space and combines it in a toaster oven with other cooking functions, like baking, broiling, toasting and sometimes rotisserie-cooking and dehydrating too. It is basically a multi-function countertop convection oven with a motorized fan on top of the unit that blows the hot air down directly on foods, rather than circulating the air around the oven cavity. It's perfect for the cook who would like to have the ability to air fry, but wants to have multiple cooking functions without sacrificing more counter space.

The Benefits of Owning the COSORI Air Fryer Oven

1. Takes Up Less Space

You don't have to worry about where to put your air fryer oven because it doesn't require much space. It is smaller compared to the convection oven. You only need around 1 foot cubed space for this kitchen device. When you are done with your air fryer oven, you can safely keep it away and bring it out the next time you want to use it. Majority of people keep their air fryer ovens on the kitchen countertops. This is something you can do if you're going to enjoy the pleasing sight of your air fryer oven.

2. Safe to Use

The process of deep frying foods has some dangers attached to it. Imagine throwing in French fries in extremely hot oil. Accidents can occur. For example, the splattering oil could burn you. Also, you can cause a fire that can destroy property or even worse, lead to death.

You don't have to worry about these unpleasant occurrences when using an air fryer because all the cooking happens inside it. The appliance is locked, and there's no splattering oil.

You can't be exposed to radiation when using air fryer like you would when using a microwave.

It gets better with air fryers. These kitchen appliances have auto shutdown. This means that the fryer turns itself off after your food is ready. Therefore, you won't have burnt food.

3. Preserves Nutrients

The process of air frying food protects the food from losing too much moisture. The fact that this method uses little oil and there's circulation of hot air creates a coating on the food. Therefore, your food will keep most of its nutrients.

If you are preparing your food with the aim of enjoying the nutrients, then an air fryer will help you to do that.

4. No Oil Smell

Most people don't like to smell like food. Imagine making delicious French fries at home and then smelling like them as you move around interacting with people.

Your entire home could also be smelling of French fries from the oil used to prepare it. This can happen if you use the normal deep fat fryer. The oil can even splatter around the kitchen increasing the concentration of the cooking smells.

The air fryer oven ensures you don't have any smells since all the oil and smells are enclosed within the appliance.

5. Cooks with Almost No Oil

We know how dangerous too much oil can be to our bodies. The air fryer oven saves us from complications arising from taking in a lot of oil. When using air fryer oven, you'll only use about 20% of the oil you normally use to cook.

There are some models that do not use any oil at all. This means that you'll take in less fat and calories which is good news if you're trying to lose weight or stay healthy. Also, you'll spend less money on cooking oil.

6. Makes Low Fat Food with Fewer Calories

If you want to take in fewer calories and fat, buy an air fryer oven. With this cooking appliance, you'll use about one tablespoon of oil or less to prepare your food.

You'll food tasty and crunchy food without adding any calories to your body. That's the perfect situation. When you deep fry foods, the food takes in a lot of oil because it has been dipped into the oil. The fact that this doesn't happen with an air fryer oven makes it possible to enjoy food with less fat and calories.

Useful Tips Before Using Your COSORI Air Fryer Tips

1. Make sure that the voltage indicated on the appliance corresponds to the local available voltage before you connect the appliance.
2. Do not use the appliance if the plug or the power cord or the appliance itself is damaged.
3. Never immerse the cord, plug, or housing, which contains electrical components and heating elements, in water or any other liquid, nor rinse under tap water. See instructions for cleaning.
4. Do not let any water or other liquid enter the appliance to prevent electric shock.
5. Always put the ingredients to be fried in the accessories included to prevent them from coming into contact with the heating elements.
6. Do not cover the air inlet and the air outlet while the appliance is operating.
7. Do not add oil to the drip tray or pans, as this may cause a fire hazard.
8. While cooking, the internal temperature of the unit reaches several hundred degrees Fahrenheit. To avoid personal injury, never place hands inside the unit unless it is thoroughly cooled.
9. Keep the power cord away from hot surfaces.
10. Do not place the appliance on or near combustible materials such as a tablecloth or curtain.
11. Use only on a level, dry, and heat-resistant surface.
12. Do not place the appliance against a wall or against other appliances. Leave at least 3.9 in. (10 cm) free space on the back, sides, and above the appliance. Do not place anything on top of the appliance.
13. Do not use the appliance for any other purpose than described in this manual.
14. WARNING: During hot air frying, hot steam is released through the air outlet openings on the back of the air fryer oven. Keep your hands and face at a safe distance from the steam and from the air outlet openings. Also be careful of hot steam and air when you open the door of the appliance.

Tips on How to Clean Built on Grease of the COSORI Air Fryer Oven

Of course even with wiping it down after every use (or you forget to wipe it down), you will inevitably get built on grease. The following is 2 Part Step to cleaning built on grease.

Cleaning Part 1: Baking Soda Paste

The first part of the deep cleaning process starts with making and applying a baking soda paste.

➢ Mix 1/4 cup Baking Soda with 2 Tbl Warm Water.
➢ Mix 1/2 cup Baking Soda with Warm Water.

Using a Paint brush or toothbrush, apply the paste to the sides, back, and ceiling of the oven. In the pictures below I only applied it to half in order to do a side by side comparison. However, you will apply the paste to the inside of the entire oven.

Things to remember when applying the paste:

1. Constantly mix the paste while applying it. The baking soda tends to separate from the water.
2. Remove the trays and the drip tray.
3. You can place a piece of parchment paper or a paper towel on the floor of the oven to help with clean up.
4. When applying the paste to the ceiling of the oven, don't apply it to any place you can't reach with a sponge to clean it off.
5. As the paste dries, it will turn bright white. You can see where you missed applying the paste and add more if needed.

Once you have applied the paste to the inside of the oven, the most important part is——

Let it sit for 12 to 24 hours!

This is the most important part. Baking soda is a basic solution and works great to cut through acidic grease. However, it is not very strong, so it needs time to work.

When you are ready to remove the paste you will need:

➢ Large bowl of water
➢ Sponge with a non-scratch scouring side (or you can use a heavy duty brillo sponge that has been used and is worn down)
➢ toothbrush
➢ straw cleaning brush
➢ Norwex cloth

As you use the sponge to remove the baking soda, constantly rinse it int he bowl of water and wring it out. Use the toothbrush and straw brush to get into the tight spaces.

Do NOT press hard while scrubbing. Just take your time. This is a slow process but worth it!

Once you have removed the baking soda, use the Norwex cloth to wipe down the sides, making sure to get off any residue that is left.

You can stop at this point, but if you are like me and want your oven to look as close to brand new as possible, then the next step is....

Cleaning Part 2: Steam Cleaning

The baking soda does a great job cutting through the first few layers of the baked on grease. To get the rest off, the best thing I have found to use is my steam cleaner. The one I recommend is the Dupray Multipurpose Steam Cleaner.

Of course I don't just use this steam cleaner for my oven. It's one of my favorite things and I use it to clean just about everything.

Use the brush end of your steam cleaner to clean the sides. The trick is to steam the grease for about 10 seconds in order to allow the hot steam to melt the grease. Then you can wipe it away.

Use the fine nozzle to get into the tight spaces like at the top edge of the Vortex Plus and the metal brackets on the Omni/Omni Plus.

The steam cleaner is also fabulous at getting in the hard to reach space where the door clips in on the Vortex Plus as well as the edge between the door and the glass on the Omni/Omni Plus.

Do NOT use the steam on the heating elements, heating coil, rotisserie knob, or on the ceiling near the fan.

BREAKFAST

Nutty Whole Wheat Muffins

Servings: 8
Cooking Time: 11 Minutes

Ingredients:

- ½ cup whole-wheat flour, plus 2 tablespoons
- ¼ cup oat bran
- 2 tablespoons flaxseed meal
- ¼ cup brown sugar
- ½ teaspoon baking soda
- ½ teaspoon baking powder
- ¼ teaspoon salt
- ½ teaspoon cinnamon
- ½ cup buttermilk
- 2 tablespoons melted butter
- 1 egg
- ½ teaspoon pure vanilla extract
- ½ cup grated carrots
- ¼ cup chopped pecans
- ¼ cup chopped walnuts
- 1 tablespoon pumpkin seeds
- 1 tablespoon sunflower seeds
- 16 foil muffin cups, paper liners removed
- cooking spray

Directions:

1. Preheat the toaster oven to 330°F.
2. In a large bowl, stir together the flour, bran, flaxseed meal, sugar, baking soda, baking powder, salt, and cinnamon.
3. In a medium bowl, beat together the buttermilk, butter, egg, and vanilla. Pour into flour mixture and stir just until dry ingredients moisten. Do not beat.
4. Gently stir in carrots, nuts, and seeds.
5. Double up the foil cups so you have 8 total and spray with cooking spray.
6. Place 4 foil cups in air fryer oven and divide half the batter among them.
7. Air-fry at 330°F for 11 minutes or until toothpick inserted in center comes out clean.
8. Repeat step 7 to cook remaining 4 muffins.

Zucchini Bread

Servings: 6
Cooking Time: 30 Minutes

Ingredients:

- 1 cup grated zucchini
- 2 tablespoons grated onion
- 2 tablespoons grated Parmesan Cheese
- ½ cup skim milk
- 1 egg
- 2 tablespoons vegetable oil
- 1½ cups unbleached flour
- 1 tablespoon baking powder
- Salt to taste

Directions:

1. Preheat the toaster oven to 375° F.
2. Stir together all the ingredients in a medium bowl until smooth. Pour the batter into an oiled or nonstick regular-size 8½ × 4½ × 2¼-inch loaf pan.
3. BAKE for 30 minutes, or until a toothpick inserted in the center comes out clean.

Baked Dutch Pancake

Servings: 2
Cooking Time: 20 Minutes

Ingredients:

- ⅓ cup whole milk, room temperature
- 2 large eggs, room temperature
- 1 tablespoon granulated sugar
- 1 teaspoon orange zest

- 1 teaspoon pure vanilla extract
- ⅛ teaspoon sea salt
- ⅛ teaspoon ground cinnamon
- ⅓ cup all-purpose flour
- 1 tablespoon unsalted butter
- Maple syrup, for serving

Directions:

1. Place the rack in position Preheat the toaster oven on BAKE to 350°F for 5 minutes.

2. In a large bowl, whisk the milk, eggs, sugar, orange zest, vanilla, salt, and cinnamon until combined. Whisk in the flour until smooth. Set aside.

3. Melt the butter in a 7-inch-round cake pan in the oven for about 2 minutes.

4. Remove the cake pan from the oven and pour in the batter.

5. Bake until puffy and golden, for about 15 minutes.

6. Serve with a drizzle of maple syrup.

Bacon Cheddar Biscuits

Servings: 6

Cooking Time: 15 Minutes

Ingredients:

- 1 cup all-purpose flour
- 1 tablespoon baking powder
- ¼ teaspoon table salt
- ¼ teaspoon smoked paprika or freshly ground black pepper
- 3 tablespoons unsalted butter
- ½ cup whole milk
- 1 cup shredded sharp cheddar cheese
- 2 tablespoons minced fresh chives
- 4 slices bacon, cooked until crisp and crumbled

Directions:

1. Preheat the toaster oven to 425°F.

2. Stir the flour, baking powder, salt, and paprika in a large bowl. Using a pastry cutter or two knives, cut the butter into the flour mixture until the mixture is crumbly throughout. Pour in the milk and gently mix until just combined. Stir in the cheese, chives, and bacon.

3. Turn the dough onto a lightly floured surface and knead lightly about 8 times. Roll the dough, using a rolling pin, until about ¾ inch thick. Cut out rounds using a 2-inch cutter. Place 1 inch apart on an ungreased 12 x 12-inch baking pan. Bake for 12 to 15 minutes or until golden brown.

Strawberry Shortcake With Buttermilk Biscuits

Servings: 8

Cooking Time: 15 Minutes

Ingredients:

- 1 quart fresh strawberries, rinsed and sliced
- 2 tablespoons sugar
- 1 tablespoon lemon juice
- Buttermilk biscuit mix:
- 2 cups unbleached flour
- 2 teaspoons baking powder
- ½ teaspoon baking soda
- Salt to taste
- ¼ cup margarine
- 1 cup low-fat buttermilk
- Vegetable oil
- Nonfat whipped topping

Directions:

1. Preheat the toaster oven to 400° F.

2. Combine the strawberries, sugar, and lemon juice in a large bowl, mixing well to blend. Set aside.

3. Combine the flour, baking powder, baking soda, and salt in a large bowl. Add the margarine, cutting it into the flour with a knife or pastry

cutter. Add just enough buttermilk so that the dough will hold together when pinched.

4. Turn the dough out onto a lightly floured surface and knead 5 or 6 times. Drop the dough from a tablespoon onto an oiled or nonstick 6½ × 10-inch baking sheet. Make 8 mounds 1½ inches across and flatten the tops with a spoon.

5. BAKE for 15 minutes, or until the biscuits are lightly browned. Cool. Spoon on the fresh strawberries. Top with nonfat whipped topping and serve.

Wild Blueberry Lemon Chia Bread

Servings: 6
Cooking Time: 27 Minutes

Ingredients:

- ¼ cup extra-virgin olive oil
- ⅓ cup plus 1 tablespoon cane sugar
- 1 large egg
- 3 tablespoons fresh lemon juice
- 1 tablespoon lemon zest
- ⅔ cup milk
- 1 cup all-purpose flour
- ¾ teaspoon baking powder
- ⅛ teaspoon salt
- 2 tablespoons chia seeds
- 1 cup frozen wild blueberries
- ⅓ cup powdered sugar
- 2 teaspoons milk

Directions:

1. Preheat the toaster oven to 310°F.
2. In a medium bowl, mix the olive oil with the sugar. Whisk in the egg, lemon juice, lemon zest, and milk; set aside.
3. In a small bowl, combine the all-purpose flour, baking powder, and salt.

4. Slowly mix the dry ingredients into the wet ingredients. Stir in the chia seeds and wild blueberries.

5. Liberally spray a 7-inch springform pan with olive-oil spray. Pour the batter into the pan and place the pan in the air fryer oven. Bake for 25 to 27 minutes, or until a toothpick inserted in the center comes out clean.

6. Remove and let cool on a wire rack for 10 minutes prior to removing from the pan.

7. Meanwhile, in a small bowl, mix the powdered sugar with the milk to create the glaze.

8. Slice and serve with a drizzle of the powdered sugar glaze.

Sheet-pan Hash Browns

Servings: 2
Cooking Time: 60 Minutes

Ingredients:

- 1½ pounds Yukon Gold potatoes, unpeeled, shredded
- 3 tablespoons extra-virgin olive oil
- ½ teaspoon table salt
- ⅛ teaspoon pepper

Directions:

1. Adjust toaster oven rack to lowest position, select air-fry or convection function, and preheat the toaster oven to 450 degrees. Place potatoes in large bowl and cover with cold water. Let sit for 5 minutes.

2. Lift potatoes out of water, one handful at a time, and transfer to colander; discard water. Rinse and dry bowl. Place half of shredded potatoes in center of clean dish towel. Gather ends of towel and twist tightly to wring out excess moisture from potatoes. Transfer dried potatoes to now-empty bowl. Repeat with remaining potatoes.

3. Add oil, salt, and pepper to potatoes and toss to combine. Distribute potatoes in even layer on small rimmed baking sheet, but do not pack down. Cook until top of potatoes is spotty brown, 30 to 40 minutes, rotating sheet halfway through baking.

4. Remove sheet from oven. Using spatula, flip hash browns in sections. Return sheet to oven and continue to cook until spotty brown and dry, 10 to 15 minutes. Season with salt and pepper to taste. Serve.

Hot Italian-style Sub

Servings:3
Cooking Time: 15 Minutes

Ingredients:
- 3 Italian-style hoagie rolls
- 3 tablespoons unsalted butter, softened
- 1 teaspoon Italian seasoning
- ½ teaspoon garlic powder
- 9 slices salami
- 12 slices pepperoni
- 3 thin slices ham
- 3 tablespoons giardiniera mix, chopped
- 6 tablespoons shredded mozzarella cheese

Directions:
1. Preheat the toaster oven to 350°F. Split the rolls lengthwise, cutting almost but not quite though the roll. Place the sandwiches in a 12 x 12-inch baking pan, side by side with the open side face up.

2. Combine the butter, Italian seasoning, and garlic powder in a small bowl. Spread evenly on the inside of the hoagie rolls.

3. Layer a third of the salami, pepperoni, and ham on each sandwich. Sprinkle with the giardiniera mix and mozzarella cheese.

4. Bake for 10 to 15 minutes or until heated through and the cheese is melted.

Grilled Dagwood

Servings: 4
Cooking Time: 20 Minutes

Ingredients:
- 4 slices whole wheat or multigrain bread
- 1 tablespoon Dijon mustard
- 2 tablespoons fresh or canned bean sprouts, washed and well drained
- 2 tablespoons chopped watercress
- 2 tablespoons chopped roasted pimientos
- 3 slices reduced-fat Swiss cheese
- 2 slices low-fat honey ham
- 2 tablespoons garlic hummus
- 6 slices sweet pickle
- 4 slices low-fat smoked turkey
- 1 tablespoon Yogurt Cheese Spread (recipe follows)
- 1 tablespoon chopped Vidalia onion
- 1 tablespoon ketchup
- 1 tablespoon pitted and chopped black olives

Directions:
1. Preheat the toaster oven to 350° F.

2. Spread the first bread slice with ½ tablespoon Dijon mustard. Add 1 tablespoon sprouts, 1 tablespoon watercress, 1 tablespoon pimientos, 1 slice Swiss cheese, and 1 slice honey ham.

3. Spread the second bread slice with ½ tablespoon Dijon mustard, turn it over, and lay it on top of the first. Spread the other side of the second slice with 1 tablespoon hummus, 1 slice honey ham, 3 pickle slices, 1 tablespoon watercress, and 2 slices smoked turkey.

4. Spread the third bread slice with the Yogurt Cheese Spread, turn it over, and lay it on top of the second slice of bread. Spread the other side of

the third slice with 1 tablespoon hummus and add the chopped onion, 1 tablespoon pimientos, 3 pickle slices, 1 slice Swiss cheese, and 2 slices smoked turkey.

5. Spread the fourth bread slice with the ketchup and add 1 tablespoon sprouts, 1 tablespoon pimientos, 1 slice Swiss cheese, and the black olives. Lift up all the other bread slices together and place this one on the bottom. Then put the slices together and wrap in aluminum foil so that the seam is on the top of the slices. Open the seam to expose the tops of the slices and place on the rack in the toaster oven, seam side up.

6. BAKE 20 minutes, or until the top is lightly browned and the cheese is melted.

Garlic Basil Bread

Servings: 6
Cooking Time: 18 Minutes

Ingredients:
- Mixture:
- 3 tablespoons olive oil
- 2 garlic cloves
- ¼ cup pine nuts (pignoli)
- ½ cup fresh basil leaves
- 2 plum tomatoes, chopped
- Salt to taste
- 1 French baguette, cut diagonally into 1-inch slices

Directions:
1. Preheat the toaster oven to 400° F.
2. Process the mixture ingredients in a blender or food processor until smooth.
3. Spread the mixture on both sides of each bread slice, reassemble into a loaf, and wrap in aluminum foil.

4. BAKE for 12 minutes, or until the bread is thoroughly heated. Peel back the aluminum foil to expose the top of the bread.

5. BAKE again for 5 minutes, or until the top is lightly browned.

Breakfast Pizza

Servings: 2
Cooking Time: 60 Minutes

Ingredients:
- 3 tablespoons extra-virgin olive oil, divided, plus extra for drizzling
- 1 recipe Classic Pizza Dough (recipe follows), room temperature
- 4 ounces whole-milk mozzarella cheese, shredded (1 cup)
- ½ ounce Parmesan cheese, grated (¼ cup)
- 2 ounces (¼ cup) cottage cheese
- ⅛ teaspoon dried oregano
- 4 ounces breakfast sausage, casings removed
- 4 large eggs
- ⅛ teaspoon table salt
- ⅛ teaspoon pepper
- 2 tablespoons minced fresh chive

Directions:
1. Coat small rimmed baking sheet with 2 tablespoons oil. Press and roll dough into 11 by 8-inch rectangle on lightly floured counter. (If dough springs back during rolling, let rest for 10 minutes before rolling again.) Transfer dough to prepared sheet and re-stretch dough into 11 by 8-inch rectangle. Brush dough evenly with 1 teaspoon oil and cover with plastic wrap. Let sit in warm spot until slightly risen, about 20 minutes.

2. Adjust toaster oven rack to lowest position and preheat the toaster oven to 450 degrees. Remove plastic and, using your fingers, make

indentations all over dough. Bake until dough has puffed slightly, 5 to 7 minutes.

3. Combine mozzarella and Parmesan in bowl. Combine cottage cheese, oregano, and remaining 2 teaspoons oil in separate bowl.

4. Remove sheet from oven and, using spatula, press down on any air bubbles. Spread cottage cheese mixture evenly over top, leaving ½-inch border around edges. Pinch sausage into dime-size pieces and arrange evenly over cottage cheese mixture. Sprinkle mozzarella mixture evenly over pizza, leaving ½-inch border. Using back of spoon, create 4 evenly spaced indentations in cheese, each about 3 inches in diameter. Crack 1 egg into each well, then sprinkle with salt and pepper.

5. Bake until crust is golden brown on bottom and eggs are just set, 9 to 10 minutes for slightly runny yolks or 11 to 12 minutes for soft but set yolks. Remove pizza from pan and transfer to wire rack; let rest for 5 minutes. Sprinkle with chives and drizzle with extra oil. Cut into 8 equal pieces and serve.

English Muffins

Servings: 2
Cooking Time: 4 Minutes

Ingredients:
- 1 English muffin, split
- 1 plum tomato, chopped
- 2 slices reduced-fat or low-fat cheese
- 2 slices reduced-fat honey ham
- 1 tablespoon chopped fresh parsley

Directions:
1. Layer each muffin half with equal portions of tomato, cheese, and ham. Place on a broiling rack with a pan underneath.

2. TOAST once.

3. Garnish each with equal portions of chopped parsley.

Blueberry Lemon Muffins

Servings: 12
Cooking Time: 23 Minutes

Ingredients:
- 2 ¼ cups all-purpose flour
- 1 ½ cups fresh blueberries
- 3/4 cup granulated sugar
- 2 teaspoons baking powder
- ½ teaspoon lemon zest
- ½ teaspoon salt
- ¾ cup milk
- ¼ cup butter, melted
- 1 tablespoon lemon juice
- 1 large egg

Directions:
1. Preheat the toaster oven to 375°F. Grease or line a 12-cup muffin pan with paper baking cups. Set aside.

2. In a large bowl, stir together flour, blueberries, granulated sugar, baking powder and salt.

3. In a small bowl, using an electric mixer or whisk, beat milk, butter, lemon juice and egg until blended.

4. Gradually add milk mixture to flour mixture. Stir until just blended.

5. Spoon into prepared muffin pan.

6. Bake 20 to 23 minutes or until toothpick inserted in center comes out clean.

Baked Grapefruit

Servings: 4
Cooking Time: 20 Minutes

Ingredients:
- 1 grapefruit, cut in half
- 2 tablespoons currant jelly

- 2 tablespoons ground almonds, walnuts, or pecans
- 2 tablespoons chopped raisins

Directions:

1. Preheat the toaster oven to 350° F.
2. Section the grapefruit halves with a serrated knife. Place them in an oiled or nonstick 8½ × 8½ × 2-inch square baking (cake) pan. Spread 1 tablespoon currant jelly on each half and sprinkle each with 1 tablespoon ground nuts and 1 tablespoon chopped raisins.
3. BAKE for 20 minutes, or until the grapefruit is lightly browned.

Portable Omelet

Servings: 1
Cooking Time: 4 Minutes

Ingredients:

- 2 slices multigrain bread
- 2 eggs
- 1 tablespoon plain nonfat yogurt
- Salt and freshly ground black pepper
- 2 strips turkey bacon
- 2 tablespoons shredded low-moisture, part-skim mozzarella cheese

Directions:

1. TOAST the bread slices and set aside.
2. Whisk together the eggs and yogurt in a small bowl and season with salt and pepper to taste.
3. Layer bacon strips in a small 4 × 8 × 2¼-inch loaf pan. Pour the egg mixture on top and sprinkle with the cheese.
4. TOAST once, or until the egg is done to your preference. Cut the omelet into toast-size squares and place between the 2 slices of toast to make a sandwich. (TOAST takes 2 to 3 minutes.)

Apple Maple Pudding

Servings: 4
Cooking Time: 20 Minutes

Ingredients:

- Pudding mixture:
- 2 eggs
- ½ cup brown sugar
- 4 tablespoons maple syrup
- 3 tablespoons unbleached flour
- 1 teaspoon baking powder
- 1 teaspoon vanilla extract
- ¼ cup chopped raisins
- ¼ cup chopped walnuts
- 2 medium apples, peeled and chopped

Directions:

1. Preheat the toaster oven to 350° F.
2. Combine the pudding mixture ingredients in a medium bowl, beating the eggs, sugar, and maple syrup together first, then adding the flour, baking powder, and vanilla. Add the raisins, nuts, and apples and mix thoroughly. Pour into an oiled or nonstick 8½ × 8½ × 2-inch square baking (cake) pan.
3. BAKE for 20 minutes, or until a toothpick inserted in the center comes out clean.
4. BROIL for 5 minutes, or until the top is lightly browned.

Best-ever Cinnamon Rolls

Servings: 10
Cooking Time: 18 Minutes

Ingredients:

- 1 tablespoon unsalted butter, softened
- DOUGH
- ½ cup whole milk
- 2 tablespoons unsalted butter, softened
- 3 tablespoons granulated sugar
- ½ teaspoon table salt

- 1 large egg
- 1 ⅔ cups all-purpose flour, plus more for kneading and dusting
- 1 ¼ teaspoons instant yeast
- FILLING
- ⅔ cup packed dark brown sugar
- 1 tablespoon plus 1 teaspoon ground cinnamon
- Pinch table salt
- 3 tablespoons unsalted butter, melted
- GLAZE
- 1 ½ cups confectioners' sugar
- 1 to 2 tablespoon whole milk
- 1 tablespoon brewed coffee
- ½ teaspoon pure vanilla extract
- 1 tablespoon unsalted butter, melted

Directions:

1. Spread the 1 tablespoon softened butter generously on the sides and bottom of an 8-inch round baking pan.

2. Combine the milk, 2 tablespoons softened butter, sugar, and salt in a 4-cup glass measuring cup. Microwave on High (100 percent) power for 40 seconds or until warm (110°F). (All the butter may not melt.) Whisk in the egg.

3. Stir the flour and yeast in a large bowl. Add the liquid ingredients and stir until you have a soft dough. Flour your hands and a clean surface. Transfer the dough to the floured surface and form it into a ball. Add flour as necessary and knead by pressing the dough with the heel of your hands and turning and repeating. Add just enough flour to keep the dough from being sticky.

4. When the dough is smooth and springs back when you press it with you finger (after 3 to 5 minutes of kneading), place the dough ball into a large oiled bowl, cover with a tea towel, and let rise in a warm place for about an hour or until the dough has almost doubled in size.

5. Transfer the dough to a floured surface and roll into a 10 x 14-inch rectangle.

6. Make the filling: Combine the brown sugar, cinnamon, and salt in a small bowl. Using a pastry brush, brush the melted butter over the entire surface of the dough. Sprinkle the cinnamon-sugar mixture over the butter, using your fingers to lightly press the mixture into the dough. Starting with the longer side, roll up the dough to form a 14-inch cylinder. Gently cut the cylinder into 10 even rolls, using a serrated knife. Place in the prepared pan, cut side up. Cover and let rise in a warm place for about 45 to 60 minutes or until doubled.

7. Preheat the toaster oven to 350°F. Bake for 16 to 18 minutes or until slightly brown on top. Remove from the oven and place on a wire rack.

8. Meanwhile, make the glaze: Whisk the confectioners' sugar, 1 tablespoon milk, the coffee, vanilla, and butter in a medium bowl. If needed, whisk in the additional milk to make the desired consistency. Drizzle over the warm rolls.

Sweet-hot Pepperoni Pizza

Servings: 2
Cooking Time: 18 Minutes

Ingredients:
- 1 (6- to 8-ounce) pizza dough ball
- olive oil
- ½ cup pizza sauce
- ¾ cup grated mozzarella cheese
- ½ cup thick sliced pepperoni
- ⅓ cup sliced pickled hot banana peppers
- ¼ teaspoon dried oregano
- 2 teaspoons honey

Directions:

1. Preheat the toaster oven to 390°F.

2. Cut out a piece of aluminum foil the same size as the bottom of the air fryer oven. Brush the foil circle with olive oil. Shape the dough into a circle and place it on top of the foil. Dock the dough by piercing it several times with a fork. Brush the dough lightly with olive oil and transfer it into the air fryer oven with the foil on the bottom.

3. Air-fry the plain pizza dough for 6 minutes. Turn the dough over, remove the aluminum foil and brush again with olive oil. Air-fry for an additional 4 minutes.

4. Spread the pizza sauce on top of the dough and sprinkle the mozzarella cheese over the sauce. Top with the pepperoni, pepper slices and dried oregano. Lower the temperature of the air fryer oven to 350°F and air-fry for 8 minutes, until the cheese has melted and lightly browned. Transfer the pizza to a cutting board and drizzle with the honey. Slice and serve.

New York–style Crumb Cake

Servings: 8

Cooking Time: 90 Minutes

Ingredients:

- CRUMB TOPPING
- 8 tablespoons unsalted butter, melted
- ⅓ cup (2⅓ ounces) granulated sugar
- ⅓ cup packed (2⅓ ounces) dark brown sugar
- ¾ teaspoon ground cinnamon
- ⅛ teaspoon table salt
- 1¾ cups (7 ounces) cake flour
- CAKE
- 1¼ cups (5 ounces) cake flour
- ½ cup (3½ ounces) granulated sugar
- ¼ teaspoon baking soda
- ¼ teaspoon table salt

- 6 tablespoons unsalted butter, cut into 6 pieces and softened
- ⅓ cup buttermilk
- 1 large egg plus 1 large yolk
- 1 teaspoon vanilla extract
- Confectioners' sugar

Directions:

1. Adjust toaster oven rack to middle position and preheat the toaster oven to 325 degrees. Make foil sling for 8-inch square baking pan by folding 2 long sheets of aluminum foil so each is 8 inches wide. Lay sheets of foil in pan perpendicular to each other, with extra foil hanging over edges of pan. Push foil into corners and up sides of pan, smoothing foil flush to pan.

2. FOR THE CRUMB TOPPING: Whisk melted butter, granulated sugar, brown sugar, cinnamon, and salt in medium bowl until combined. Add flour and stir with rubber spatula or wooden spoon until mixture resembles thick, cohesive dough; set aside to cool to room temperature, 10 to 15 minutes.

3. FOR THE CAKE: Using stand mixer fitted with paddle, mix flour, sugar, baking soda, and salt on low speed to combine. With mixer running, add softened butter 1 piece at a time. Continue beating until mixture resembles moist crumbs with no visible butter pieces remaining, 1 to 2 minutes. Add buttermilk, egg and yolk, and vanilla and beat on medium-high speed until light and fluffy, about 1 minute, scraping down bowl as needed.

4. Transfer batter to prepared pan. Using rubber spatula, spread batter into even layer. Break apart crumb topping into large pea-size pieces and sprinkle in even layer over batter, beginning with edges and then working toward center. (Assembled cake can be wrapped tightly with

plastic wrap and refrigerated for up to 24 hours; increase baking time to 40 to 45 minutes.)

5. Bake until crumbs are golden and toothpick inserted in center of cake comes out clean, 35 to 40 minutes, rotating pan halfway through baking. Let cool on wire rack for at least 30 minutes. Using foil overhang, lift cake out of pan. Dust with confectioners' sugar before serving.

Baked Eggs And Bacon

Servings: 2
Cooking Time: 25 Minutes

Ingredients:
- 8 slices bacon
- 4 large eggs
- 2 teaspoons fresh chives or scallion greens, chopped
- Sea salt, for seasoning
- Freshly ground black pepper, for seasoning

Directions:
1. Place the baking tray on position 1 and preheat the toaster oven on BAKE to 400°F for 5 minutes.
2. Arrange the bacon slices in four (4-ounce) ramekins, 2 per cup. Overlap the slices over the bottom and sides so that as much of the cup is covered as possible.
3. Bake for 10 to 15 minutes. The fat will start to render, and the bacon will start to crisp and brown on the edges. Take the ramekins out of the oven and lightly blot any excess oil in the bottom of each one.
4. Crack 1 egg into each cup, sprinkle with chives, and season lightly with salt and pepper.
5. Bake for 10 minutes, or until the egg yolks reach the desired consistency.

6. Take them out of the oven and run a knife around the edge of each cup to loosen and remove from the ramekin. Serve.

Broiled Grapefruit With Cinnamon Brown Sugar

Servings: 4
Cooking Time: 7 Minutes

Ingredients:
- 2 large grapefruit, halved
- 1/4 cup packed light brown sugar
- 1/4 teaspoon ground cinnamon
- 1 tablespoon butter, softened
- 1/4 cup vanilla yogurt
- 2 tablespoons granola

Directions:
1. Preheat the toaster oven to 400°F. Place rack in upper position.
2. Remove all seeds from grapefruit and section with a paring knife. Cut a small slice from the bottom of each grapefruit half to prevent them from rocking. Place grapefruit halves on toaster oven baking pan.
3. In small bowl, mix brown sugar and cinnamon. Sprinkle evenly over top of grapefruit halves. Dot with butter.
4. Broil for 6 to 7 minutes or until brown sugar and butter is bubbly. Top each half with 1 tablespoon yogurt and 1/2 tablespoon granola.

Popovers

Servings: 6
Cooking Time: 30 Minutes

Ingredients:
- 2 eggs
- 1 cup skim milk
- 2 tablespoons vegetable oil
- 1 cup unbleached flour

- Salt to taste

Directions:
1. Preheat the toaster oven to 400° F.
2. Beat all the ingredients in a medium bowl with an electric mixer at high speed until smooth. The batter should be the consistency of heavy cream.
3. Fill the pans of a 6-muffin tin three-quarters full.
4. BAKE for 20 minutes, then reduce the heat to 350° F. and bake for 10 minutes, or until golden brown.

Flaky Granola

Servings: 3
Cooking Time: 20 Minutes

Ingredients:
- ¼ cup rolled oats
- ½ cup wheat flakes
- ½ cup bran flakes
- ¼ cup wheat germ
- 3 tablespoons sesame seeds
- 4 ¼ cup unsweetened shredded coconut
- ½ cup chopped almonds, walnuts, or pecans
- 2 tablespoons chopped pumpkin seeds
- ½ cup honey or molasses
- 2 tablespoons vegetable oil
- Salt to taste

Directions:
1. Preheat the toaster oven to 375° F.
2. Combine all the ingredients in a medium bowl, stirring to mix well.
3. Spread the mixture in an oiled or nonstick 6½ × 6½ × 2-inch square (cake) pan.
4. BAKE for 20 minutes, turning with tongs every 5 minutes to toast evenly. Cool and store in an airtight container in the refrigerator.

Buttermilk Biscuits

Servings: 6
Cooking Time: 15minutes

Ingredients:
- 2 cups unbleached flour
- 1 tablespoon baking powder
- ½ teaspoon baking soda
- Salt
- 3 tablespoons margarine, at room temperature
- 1 cup low-fat buttermilk
- Vegetable oil

Directions:
1. Preheat the toaster oven to 400° F.
2. Combine the flour, baking powder, baking soda, and salt to taste in a medium bowl.
3. Cut in the margarine with 2 knives or a pastry blender until the mixture is crumbly.
4. Stir in the buttermilk, adding just enough so the dough will stay together when pinched.
5. KNEAD the dough on a floured surface for one minute, then pat or roll out the dough to ¾ inch thick. Cut out biscuit rounds with a 2½-inch biscuit cutter. Place the rounds on an oiled or nonstick 6½ × 10inch baking sheet.
6. BAKE for 15 minutes, or until golden brown.

Cinnamon Toast

Servings: 2
Cooking Time: 2 Minutes

Ingredients:
- 1 tablespoon brown sugar
- 2 teaspoons margarine, at room temperature
- ¼ teaspoon ground cinnamon
- 2 slices whole wheat or multigrain bread

Directions:
1. Combine the sugar, margarine, and cinnamon in a small bowl with a fork until well blended.

Spread each bread slice with equal portions of the mixture.

2. TOAST once, or until the sugar is melted and the bread is browned to your preference.

Apple Incredibles

Servings: 6
Cooking Time: 25 Minutes

Ingredients:
- Muffin mixture:
- 2 cups unbleached flour
- 1 teaspoon baking powder
- ¼ cup brown sugar
- ½ teaspoon salt
- ¼ cup margarine, at room temperature
- ½ cup skim milk
- 1 egg, beaten
- 2 tablespoons finely chopped raisins
- 2 tablespoons finely chopped pecans
- 1 apple, peeled, cored, and thinly sliced

Directions:
1. Preheat the toaster oven to 400° F.
2. Combine the muffin mixture ingredients in a large bowl, stirring just to blend. Fill the pans of an oiled or nonstick 6-muffin tin with the batter. Insert the apple slices vertically into the batter, standing and pushing them all the way down to the bottom of the pan.
3. BAKE for 25 minutes, or until the apples are tender and the muffins are lightly browned.

LUNCH AND DINNER

Homemade Beef Enchiladas

Servings: 4
Cooking Time: 20 Minutes

Ingredients:

- 1 tablespoon canola or vegetable oil
- 1 tablespoon plus 1 teaspoon all-purpose flour
- 2 tablespoons chili powder
- ½ teaspoon ground cumin
- ½ teaspoon garlic powder
- ¼ teaspoon kosher salt
- 1 ¼ cups chicken or vegetable broth
- ¾ pound lean ground beef
- Nonstick cooking spray
- 8 flour or corn tortillas
- ¼ cup finely chopped onion
- 1 ½ cups shredded Mexican-blend or cheddar cheese

Directions:

1. Heat the oil in a small saucepan over medium-high heat. Add the flour and whisk for about a minute. Stir in the chili powder, cumin, garlic powder, and salt. Gradually stir in the broth, whisking until smooth. Reduce the heat to a simmer and cook the sauce for 10 to 12 minutes.

2. Cook the ground beef in a medium skillet over medium-high heat until browned and cooked through, stirring to crumble into a fine texture. Remove from the heat and drain.

3. Preheat the toaster oven to 350°F. Spray an 11 x 7 x 2 ½-inch baking dish with nonstick cooking spray. Place about ½ cup sauce over the bottom of the dish. Lay a tortilla on a large plate and spread about 2 tablespoons of sauce over the surface of the tortilla. Spoon 2 tablespoons of the ground beef down the center of the tortilla.

Sprinkle with some onion and cheese (amount is up to you). Roll up and place in the baking dish. Repeat with the remaining tortillas. Pour the remaining sauce over the top. Sprinkle with remaining cheese. Bake, uncovered, for 20 minutes or until the tortillas are heated through and slightly crisp on the outside.

Glazed Pork Tenderloin With Carrots Sheet Pan Supper

Servings: 4-6
Cooking Time: 20 Minutes

Ingredients:

- 1 pound pork tenderloin
- 1 teaspoon steak seasoning blend
- 2 large carrots, sliced 1/2-inch thick
- 2 large parsnips, sliced 1/2-inch thick
- 1/2 small sweet onion, cut in thin wedges
- 1 tablespoon olive oil
- Salt and pepper to taste
- 1/2 cup apricot jam
- 1 tablespoon balsamic vinegar

Directions:

1. Place rack on bottom position of toaster oven. Heat the toaster oven to 425°F. Spray the toaster oven baking pan with nonstick cooking spray or line the pan with nonstick aluminum foil.

2. Place pork tenderloin diagonally in center of pan. Sprinkle pork with seasoning blend.

3. In a large bowl, combine carrots, parsnips and onion. Add olive oil, salt and black pepper and stir until vegetables are coated. Arrange vegetables evenly in pan around pork.

4. Bake 20 minutes. Stir vegetables.

5. Meanwhile, in a small bowl, combine apricot jam and balsamic vinegar. Spoon about half of mixture over pork.

6. Continue baking until pork reaches reaches 160°F when tested with a meat thermometer and vegetables are roasted, about 10 minutes. Slice pork and serve with remaining sauce, if desired.

One-step Classic Goulash

Servings: 4
Cooking Time: 56 Minutes

Ingredients:
- 1 cup elbow macaroni
- 1 cup (8-ounce can) tomato sauce
- 1 cup very lean ground round or sirloin
- 1 cup peeled and chopped fresh tomato
- ½ cup finely chopped onion
- 1 teaspoon garlic powder
- Salt and freshly ground black pepper
- Topping:
- 1 cup homemade bread crumbs
- 1 tablespoon margarine

Directions:
1. Preheat the toaster oven to 400° F.
2. Combine all the ingredients, except the topping, with 2 cups water in a 1-quart 8½ × 8½ × 4-inch ovenproof baking dish and mix well. Adjust the seasonings to taste. Cover with aluminum foil.
3. BAKE, covered, for 50 minutes, or until the macaroni is cooked, stirring after 25 minutes to distribute the liquid. Uncover, sprinkle with bread crumbs, and dot with margarine.
4. BROIL for 6 minutes, or until the topping is lightly browned.

Italian Bread Pizza

Servings: 4

Cooking Time: 30 Minutes

Ingredients:
- 1 loaf Italian or French bread, unsliced
- Filling:
- ½ cup tomato sauce
- 2 tablespoons tomato paste
- 2 tablespoons olive oil
- ½ cup grated zucchini
- ½ cup grated onion
- 2 tablespoons grated bell pepper
- 1 teaspoon garlic powder
- 2 tablespoons chopped pitted black olives
- 1 teaspoon dried oregano or 1 tablespoon chopped fresh oregano
- Salt to taste
- ¼ cup mozzarella cheese

Directions:
1. Preheat the toaster oven to 375° F.
2. Cut the loaf of bread in half lengthwise, then in quarters crosswise. Remove some of the bread from the center to make a cavity for the pizza topping.
3. Combine all the topping ingredients and spoon equal portions into the cavities in the bread. Sprinkle with mozzarella cheese. Place the bread quarters on the toaster oven rack.
4. BAKE for 30 minutes, or until the cheese is melted and the crust is lightly browned.

Sage, Chicken + Mushroom Pasta Casserole

Servings: 6
Cooking Time: 35 Minutes

Ingredients:
- Nonstick cooking spray
- 8 ounces bow-tie pasta, uncooked
- 4 tablespoons unsalted butter
- 8 ounces button or white mushrooms, sliced

- 3 tablespoons all-purpose flour
- Kosher salt and freshly ground black pepper
- 2 cups whole milk
- ½ cup dry white wine
- 2 tablespoons minced fresh sage
- 1 ½ cups chopped cooked chicken
- 1 cup shredded fontina, Monterey Jack, or Swiss cheese
- ½ cup shredded Parmesan cheese

Directions:

1. Preheat the toaster oven to 350°F. Spray a 2-quart baking pan with nonstick cooking spray.
2. Cook the pasta according to the package directions; drain and set aside.
3. Melt the butter in a large skillet over medium-high heat. Add the mushrooms and cook, stirring frequently, until the liquid has evaporated, 7 to 10 minutes. Blend in the flour and cook, stirring constantly, for 1 minute. Season with salt and pepper. Gradually stir in the milk and wine. Cook, stirring constantly, until the mixture bubbles and begins to thicken. Remove from the heat. Stir in the sage, cooked pasta, chicken, and fontina. Season with salt and pepper.
4. Spoon into the prepared pan. Cover and bake for 25 to 30 minutes. Uncover, sprinkle with the Parmesan, and bake for an additional 5 minutes or until the cheese is melted.
5. Remove from the oven and let stand for 5 to 10 minutes before serving.

Gardener's Rice

Servings: 4
Cooking Time: 40 Minutes

Ingredients:
- ½ cup rice
- 2 tablespoons finely chopped scallions

- 2 small zucchini, finely chopped
- 1 bell pepper, finely chopped
- 1 small tomato, finely chopped
- ¼ cup frozen peas
- ¼ cup frozen corn
- 1 teaspoon ground cumin
- ½ teaspoon dried oregano or
- 1 teaspoon chopped fresh oregano
- Salt and freshly ground black pepper to taste

Directions:

1. Preheat the toaster oven to 400° F.
2. Combine all the ingredients with ¼ cups water in a 1-quart 8½ × 8½ × 4-inch ovenproof baking dish, stirring well to blend. Adjust the seasonings to taste. Cover with aluminum foil.
3. BAKE, covered, for 30 minutes, or until the rice and vegetables are almost cooked. Remove from the oven, uncover, and let stand for 10 minutes to complete the cooking. Fluff once more and adjust the seasonings before serving.

Kasha Loaf

Servings: 4
Cooking Time: 30 Minutes

Ingredients:
- 1 cup whole grain kasha
- 2 cups tomato sauce or 3 2 8-ounce cans tomato sauce (add a small amount of water to make 4 2 cups)
- 3 tablespoons minced onion or scallions
- 1 tablespoon minced garlic
- 1 cup multigrain bread crumbs
- 1 egg
- 1 teaspoon paprika
- 1 teaspoon chili powder
- 1 teaspoon sesame oil

Directions:

1. Preheat the toaster oven to 400° F.

2. Combine all the ingredients in a bowl and transfer to an oiled or nonstick regular-size 4½ × 8½ × 2/4-inch loaf pan.

3. BAKE, uncovered, for 30 minutes, or until lightly browned.

Easy Oven Lasagne

Servings: 4
Cooking Time: 60 Minutes

Ingredients:
- 6 uncooked lasagna noodles, broken in half
- 1 15-ounce jar marinara sauce
- ½ pound ground turkey or chicken breast
- ½ cup part-skim ricotta cheese
- ½ cup shredded part-skim mozzarella cheese
- 2 tablespoons chopped fresh oregano leaves or 1 teaspoon dried oregano
- 2 tablespoons chopped fresh basil leaves or 1 teaspoon dried basil
- 1 tablespoon garlic cloves, minced
- ¼ cup grated Parmesan cheese
- Salt and freshly ground black pepper to taste

Directions:
1. Preheat the toaster oven to 375° F.

2. Layer in a 1-quart 8½ × 8½ × 4-inch ovenproof baking dish in this order: 6 lasagna noodle halves, ½ jar of the marinara sauce, ½ cup water, half of the ground meat, half of the ricotta and mozzarella cheeses, half of the oregano and basil leaves, and half of the minced garlic. Repeat the layer, starting with the noodles. Cover the dish with aluminum foil.

3. BAKE, covered, for 50 minutes, or until the noodles are tender. Uncover, sprinkle the top with Parmesan cheese and bake for another 10 minutes, or until the liquid is reduced and the top is browned.

Narragansett Clam Chowder

Servings: 4
Cooking Time: 35 Minutes

Ingredients:
- 1 cup fat-free half-and-half
- 2 tablespoons unbleached flour
- 3 ½ cup chopped onion
- 1 cup peeled and diced potato
- 1 tablespoon vegetable oil
- 1 tablespoon chopped fresh parsley
- 1 6-ounce can clams, drained and chopped
- 1 15-ounce can fat-free low-sodium chicken broth
- Salt and freshly ground black pepper

Directions:
1. Whisk together the half-and-half and flour in a small bowl. Set aside.

2. Combine the onion, potato, and oil in an 8½ × 8½ × 2-inch square baking (cake) pan.

3. BROIL 15 minutes, turning every 5 minutes with tongs, or until the potato is tender and the onion is cooked. Transfer to a 1-quart baking dish. Add the parsley, clams, broth, and half-and-half/flour mixture. Stir well and season to taste with salt and pepper.

4. BAKE, uncovered, at 375° F. for 20 minutes, stirring after 10 minutes, or until the stock is reduced and thickened. Ladle into bowls and serve with Yogurt Bread.

Yeast Dough For Two Pizzas

Servings: 8
Cooking Time: 20 Minutes

Ingredients:
- ¼ cup tepid water
- 1 cup tepid skim milk
- ½ teaspoon sugar
- 1 1¼-ounce envelope dry yeast

- 2 cups unbleached flour
- 1 tablespoon olive oil

Directions:

1. Preheat the toaster oven to 400° F.

2. Combine the water, milk, and sugar in a bowl. Add the yeast and set aside for 3 to 5 minutes, or until the yeast is dissolved.

3. Stir in the flour gradually, adding just enough to form a ball of the dough.

4. KNEAD on a floured surface until the dough is satiny, and then put the dough in a bowl in a warm place with a damp towel over the top. In 1 hour or when the dough has doubled in bulk, punch it down and divide it in half. Flatten the dough and spread it out to the desired thickness on an oiled or nonstick 9¾-inch-diameter pie pan. Spread with Homemade Pizza Sauce (recipe follows) and add any desired toppings.

5. BAKE for 20 minutes, or until the topping ingredients are cooked and the cheese is melted.

Harvest Chicken And Rice Casserole

Servings: 4
Cooking Time: 42 Minutes

Ingredients:

- 4 skinless, boneless chicken thighs, cut into 1-inch cubes
- ½ cup brown rice 4 scallions, chopped
- 1 plum tomato, chopped
- 1 cup frozen peas
- 1 cup frozen corn
- 1 cup peeled and chopped carrots
- 2 tablespoons chopped fresh parsley
- 1 teaspoon mustard seed
- 1 teaspoon dried dill weed
- ¼ teaspoon celery seed
- Salt and freshly ground black pepper to taste

- ½ cup finely chopped pecans

Directions:

1. Preheat the toaster oven to 400° F.

2. Combine all the ingredients, except the pecans, with 2½ cups water in a 1-quart 8½ × 8½ × 4-inch ovenproof baking dish. Adjust the seasonings to taste. Cover with aluminum foil.

3. BAKE, covered, for 45 minutes, or until the rice is tender, stirring after 20 minutes to distribute the liquid. When done, uncover and sprinkle the top with the pecans.

4. BROIL for 7 minutes, or until the pecans are browned.

Cornucopia Casserole

Servings: 4
Cooking Time: 45 Minutes

Ingredients:

- 1 celery stalk, chopped
- 2 tablespoons chopped Vidalia onion
- 3 ½ bell pepper, chopped
- 1 carrot, peeled and chopped
- 1 small zucchini, chopped
- ½ cup green beans, cut into 1-inch Pieces
- ½ cup frozen peas ½ cup frozen corn
- ½ cup frozen broccoli florets
- ½ cup frozen cauliflower florets
- 2 tablespoons vegetable oil
- 1 teaspoon ground cumin
- 1 teaspoon garlic powder
- ½ teaspoon paprika
- Salt and freshly ground black pepper to taste
- ½ cup finely chopped pecans
- 3 tablespoons grated Parmesan cheese

Directions:

1. Preheat the toaster oven to 400° F.

2. Combine all the ingredients, except the pecans and Parmesan cheese, in a 1-quart 8½ ×

8½ × 4-inch ovenproof baking dish and adjust the seasonings to taste. Cover with aluminum foil.

3. BAKE, covered, for 35 minutes, or until the vegetables are tender. Uncover, stir to distribute the liquid, and adjust the seasonings again. Sprinkle the top with the pecans and Parmesan cheese.

4. BROIL for 10 minutes, or until the pecans are lightly browned.

Crunchy Baked Chicken Tenders

Servings: 3-4
Cooking Time: 18 Minutes

Ingredients:
- 2/3 cup seasoned panko breadcrumbs
- 2/3 cup cheese crackers, crushed
- 2 teaspoons melted butter
- 2 large eggs, beaten
- Salt and pepper
- 1 1/2 pounds chicken tenders
- Barbecue sauce

Directions:
1. Preheat the toaster oven to 450°F. Spray the toaster oven baking pan with nonstick cooking spray.
2. In medium bowl, combine breadcrumbs, cheese cracker crumbs and butter.
3. In another medium bowl, mix eggs, salt and pepper.
4. Dip chicken tenders in eggs and dredge in breadcrumb mixture.
5. Place on pan.
6. Bake for 15 to 18 minutes, turning once. Serve with barbecue sauce for dipping.

Parmesan Crusted Tilapia

Servings: 2
Cooking Time: 14 Minutes

Ingredients:
- 2 ounces Parmesan cheese
- 1/4 cup Italian seasoned Panko bread crumbs
- 1/2 teaspoon Italian seasoning
- 1/4 teaspoon ground black pepper
- 1 tablespoon mayonnaise
- 2 tilapia fillets or other white fish fillets (about 4 ounces each)

Directions:
1. Preheat the toaster oven to 425°F. Spray baking pan with nonstick cooking spray.
2. Using a spiralizer, grate Parmesan cheese and place in a large resealable plastic bag. Add Panko bread crumbs, Italian seasoning and black pepper. Seal and shake bag.
3. Spread mayonnaise on both sides of fish fillets. Add fish to bag and shake until coated with crumb mixture.
4. Press remaining crumbs from bag onto fish. Place on prepared baking pan.
5. Bake until fish flakes easily with a fork, 12 to 14 minutes.

Italian Baked Stuffed Tomatoes

Servings: 4
Cooking Time: 30 Minutes

Ingredients:
- 4 large tomatoes
- 1 cup shredded chicken
- 1 1/2 cup shredded mozzarella, divided
- 1 1/2 cup cooked rice
- 2 tablespoon minced onion
- 1/4 cup grated parmesan cheese
- 1 tablespoon dried Italian seasoning
- salt
- pepper
- Basil

Directions:

1. Preheat the toaster oven to 350°F. Spray toaster oven pan with nonstick cooking spray.

2. Cut the top off each tomato and scoop centers out. Place bottoms on prepared pan. Chop 3 tomatoes (about 1 1/2 cup, chopped) and add to large bowl.

3. Add shredded chicken, 1 cup shredded mozzarella cheese, rice, onion, Parmesan cheese, Italian seasoning, salt and pepper to large bowl and stir until blended. Divide between tomatoes, about 1 cup per tomato. Top with remaining mozzarella and tomato top.

4. Bake 25 to 30 minutes until cheese is melted and mixture is heated through.

5. Garnish with basil before serving.

Pesto Pizza

Servings: 1
Cooking Time: 20 Minutes

Ingredients:
- Topping:
- ½ cup chopped fresh basil
- 1 tablespoon pine nuts (pignoli)
- 1 tablespoon olive oil
- 2 tablespoons shredded Parmesan cheese
- 1 garlic clove, minced
- ½ teaspoon dried oregano or 1 tablespoon chopped fresh oregano
- 1 plum tomato, chopped
- Salt and pepper to taste
- 1 9-inch ready-made pizza crust
- 2 tablespoons shredded low-fat mozzarella

Directions:
1. Preheat the toaster oven to 375° F.

2. Combine the topping ingredients in a small bowl.

3. Process the mixture in a blender or food processor until smooth. Spread the mixture on the pizza crust, then sprinkle with the mozzarella cheese. Place the pizza crust on the toaster oven rack.

4. BAKE for 20 minutes, or until the cheese is melted and the crust is brown.

Green Bean Soup

Servings: 4
Cooking Time: 47 Minutes

Ingredients:
- Roux mixture:
- 2 tablespoons unbleached flour
- 1 tablespoon margarine
- 3 cups water or low-sodium vegetable stock
- 1 cup (½ pound) fresh string beans, trimmed and cut into 1-inch pieces
- ½ teaspoon dried oregano
- ½ teaspoon ground cumin
- Salt and freshly ground black pepper to taste

Directions:
1. Combine the roux mixture in an 8½ × 8½ × 2-inch baking (cake) pan.

2. BROIL for 5 minutes, or until the margarine is melted. Remove from the oven and stir, then broil again for 2 minutes, or until the mixture is brown but not burned. Remove from the oven and stir to mix well. Set aside.

3. Combine the water or broth, string beans, and seasonings in a 1-quart 8½ × 8½ × 4-inch ovenproof baking dish. Stir in the roux mixture, blending well. Adjust the seasonings to taste.

4. BAKE, covered, at 375°F. for 40 minutes, or until the string beans are tender.

Light Beef Stroganoff

Servings: 4

Cooking Time: 40 Minutes

Ingredients:
- Sauce:
- 1 cup skim milk
- 1 cup fat-free half-and-half
- 2 tablespoons reduced-fat cream cheese, at room temperature
- 4 tablespoons unbleached flour
- 2 pounds lean round or sirloin steak, cut into strips 2 inches long and ½ inch thick
- Browning mixture:
- 1 tablespoon soy sauce
- 2 tablespoons spicy brown mustard
- 1 tablespoon olive oil
- 2 teaspoons garlic powder
- Salt and freshly ground black pepper to taste

Directions:

1. Whisk together the sauce ingredients in a medium bowl until smooth. Set aside.

2. Combine the beef strips and browning mixture ingredients in an oiled or nonstick 8½ × 8½ × 2-inch square baking (cake) pan.

3. BROIL for 8 minutes, or until the strips are browned, turning with tongs after 4 minutes. Transfer to a 1-quart 8½ × 8½ × 4-inch ovenproof baking dish. Add the sauce and mix well. Adjust the seasonings to taste. Cover with aluminum foil.

4. BAKE, covered, for 40 minutes, or until the meat is tender.

Sheet Pan Beef Fajitas

Servings: 3

Cooking Time: 10 Minutes

Ingredients:
- Nonstick cooking spray
- 3 tablespoons olive oil
- 1 ½ teaspoons chili powder
- 2 teaspoons ground cumin
- 1 teaspoon kosher salt
- 1 onion, halved and sliced into ¼-inch strips
- 1 large red or green bell pepper, cut into thin strips
- ¾-pound flank steak, cut across the grain into thin strips
- 3 tablespoons fresh lime juice
- 3 cloves garlic, minced
- 6 flour or corn tortillas, warmed

Directions:

1. Position the rack to broil. Preheat the toaster oven on the Broil setting. Spray a 12 x 12-inch baking pan with nonstick cooking spray.

2. Combine the olive oil, chili powder, cumin, and salt in a small bowl. Add the onion and bell pepper and toss to coat them evenly with the mixture. Use a slotted spoon to remove the vegetables from the seasoned oil mixture. Reserve the seasoned oil mixture. Place the vegetables in a single layer on the prepared pan. Broil for about 5 minutes or until the vegetables are beginning to brown.

3. Meanwhile, toss the steak strips in the reserved seasoned oil mixture. Push the vegetables to one side of the pan and add the steak in a single layer on the other side of the pan. Broil for 5 minutes.

4. When the meat is done, remove the meat from the pan and toss with the lime juice and garlic. Serve the meat and vegetables in warm tortillas.

Spanako Pizza

Servings: 2
Cooking Time: 30 Minutes

Ingredients:

- 8 sheets phyllo dough, thawed and folded in half
- 4 tablespoons olive oil
- 4 tablespoons grated Parmesan cheese
- Topping mixture:
- 1 10-ounce package frozen chopped spinach, thawed and well drained
- 1 plum tomato, finely chopped
- ¼ cup finely chopped onion
- ¼ cup shredded low-fat mozzarella cheese
- 3 tablespoons crumbled feta cheese or part-skim ricotta cheese
- 2 garlic cloves, minced
- Salt and freshly ground black pepper to taste

Directions:

1. Preheat the toaster oven to 375° F.
2. Layer the sheets of phyllo dough in an oiled or nonstick 9¾-inch-diameter baking pan, lightly brushing the top of each sheet with olive oil and folding in the corner edges to fit the pan.
3. Combine the topping mixture ingredients in a bowl and adjust the seasonings to taste. Spread the mixture on top of the phyllo pastry layers and sprinkle with the Parmesan cheese.
4. BAKE for 30 minutes, or until the cheese is melted and the topping is lightly browned. Remove carefully from the pan with a metal spatula.

Miso-glazed Salmon With Broccoli

Servings: 2
Cooking Time: 25 Minutes

Ingredients:

- Nonstick cooking spray
- 2 tablespoons miso, preferably yellow
- 2 tablespoons mirin
- 1 tablespoon packed dark brown sugar
- 2 teaspoons minced fresh ginger
- 1 ½ teaspoons sesame oil
- 8 ounces fresh broccoli, cut into spears
- 1 tablespoon canola or vegetable oil
- Kosher salt and freshly ground black pepper
- 2 salmon fillets (5 to 6 ounces each)

Directions:

1. Preheat the toaster oven to 425°F. Spray a 12 x 12-inch baking pan with nonstick cooking spray.
2. Stir the miso, mirin, brown sugar, ginger, and sesame oil in a small bowl; set aside.
3. Toss the broccoli spears with the canola oil and season with salt and pepper. Place the broccoli on the pan. Bake, uncovered, for 10 minutes. Stir the broccoli and move to one side of the pan.
4. Place the salmon, skin side down, on the other end of the pan. Brush lightly with olive oil and season with salt and pepper. Bake for 10 minutes.
5. Brush the fish generously with the miso sauce. Bake for an additional 3 to 5 minutes, or until the fish flakes easily with a fork and a meat thermometer registers 145°F.

Tarragon Beef Ragout

Servings: 6
Cooking Time: 53 Minutes

Ingredients:

- 1 pound lean round steak, cut across the grain of the meat into thin strips, approximately ¼ × 2 inches
- ½ cup dry red wine

- 1 small onion, chopped
- 2 carrots, peeled and thinly sliced
- 3 2 plum tomatoes, chopped
- 1 celery stalk, chopped
- 1 10-ounce package frozen peas
- 3 garlic gloves, minced
- 1 tablespoon Dijon mustard
- ½ teaspoon ground cumin
- ½ teaspoon dried tarragon
- Salt and freshly ground black pepper to taste

Directions:

1. Preheat the toaster oven to 375° F.
2. Combine all the ingredients with ½ cup water in an 8½ × 8½ × 4-inch ovenproof baking dish. Adjust the seasonings. Cover with aluminum foil.
3. BAKE, covered, for 45 minutes, or until the beef, onion, and celery are tender. Remove the cover.
4. BROIL 8 minutes to reduce the liquid and lightly brown the top.

Sheet Pan Loaded Nachos

Servings: 4
Cooking Time: 13 Minutes

Ingredients:

- 1 tablespoon canola or vegetable oil
- ½ pound lean ground beef
- ½ cup chopped onion
- 2 cloves garlic, minced
- 1 teaspoon chili powder
- ½ teaspoon ground cumin
- Kosher salt and freshly ground black pepper
- 6 ounces tortilla chips
- ½ cup canned black beans, rinsed and drained
- 1 ½ cups shredded sharp cheddar cheese or Mexican blend cheese
- ½ cup salsa

- Optional toppings: sliced jalapeño peppers, chopped bell peppers, sliced ripe olives, chopped tomatoes, minced fresh cilantro, sour cream, chopped avocado, guacamole, or chopped onion.

Directions:

1. Preheat the toaster oven to 400°F. Line a 12 x 12-inch baking pan with nonstick aluminum foil. (Or if lining the pan with regular foil, spray it with nonstick cooking spray.)
2. Heat the oil in a large skillet over medium-high heat. Add the ground beef and onion and cook, stirring frequently, until the beef is almost done. Add the garlic, chili powder, cumin, season with salt and pepper, and cook, stirring frequently, until the beef is fully cooked; drain.
3. Arrange the tortilla chips in an even layer in the prepared pan. Top with the beef-onion mixture, then top with the beans. Bake, uncovered, for 6 to 8 minutes. Top with the cheese and bake for 5 minutes more, or until the cheese is melted.
4. Drizzle with the salsa. Top as desired with any of the various toppings.

Family Favorite Pizza

Servings: 6
Cooking Time: 22 Minutes

Ingredients:

- CRUST
- ½ cup warm water (about 110 ºF)
- 1 teaspoon active dry yeast
- 1 ½ cups all-purpose flour, plus more for kneading
- 1 teaspoon kosher salt
- ½ teaspoon olive oil
- TOPPINGS
- Pizza sauce

- 2 cups shredded Italian blend cheese or mozzarella cheese
- ¼ cup grated Parmesan cheese
- Optional toppings: pepperoni slices, cooked crumbled or sliced sausage, vegetables, or other favorite pizza toppings

Directions:

1. Make the Crust: Pour the water into a medium bowl and sprinkle with the yeast. Let stand for 5 minutes until the yeast is foamy. Add the flour, salt, and olive oil. Mix until a dough forms. Turn the dough out on a floured surface and knead until a ball forms that springs back when you poke a finger into it, about 5 minutes. If the dough is too sticky, add a tablespoon of flour and knead into the dough. Cover the dough and allow to rest for 10 minutes.

2. Preheat the toaster oven to 450°F. Place a 12-inch pizza pan in the toaster oven while it is preheating.

3. Stretch and roll the dough into an 11 ½-inch round. If the dough starts to shrink back, let it rest for 5 to 10 more minutes and then continue to roll. Carefully remove the hot pan from the toaster oven and place the pizza crust on the hot pan. Top with the desired amount of sauce. Layer cheese and any of your favorite pizza toppings over the pizza.

4. Bake for 18 to 22 minutes, or until the crust is golden brown and the cheese is melted. Let stand for 5 minutes before cutting.

Oven-baked Couscous

Servings: 4
Cooking Time: 10 Minutes

Ingredients:

- 1 10-ounce package couscous
- 2 tablespoons olive oil
- 2 tablespoons canned chickpeas
- 2 tablespoons canned or frozen green peas
- 1 tablespoon chopped fresh parsley
- 3 scallions, chopped
- Salt and pepper to taste

Directions:

1. Preheat the toaster oven to 400° F.

2. Mix together all the ingredients with 2 cups water in a 1-quart 8½ × 8½ × 4-inch ovenproof baking dish. Adjust the seasonings to taste. Cover with aluminum foil.

3. BAKE, covered, for 10 minutes, or until the couscous and vegetables are tender. Adjust the seasonings to taste and fluff with a fork before serving.

Honey Bourbon–glazed Pork Chops With Sweet Potatoes + Apples

Servings: 2
Cooking Time: 42 Minutes

Ingredients:

- Nonstick cooking spray
- 2 medium sweet potatoes, peeled and quartered
- 2 tablespoons bourbon
- 2 tablespoons honey
- 1 tablespoon canola or vegetable oil
- ½ teaspoon onion powder
- ½ teaspoon dry mustard
- ¼ teaspoon dried thyme leaves
- Kosher salt and freshly ground black pepper
- 2 bone-in pork chops, cut about ¾ inch thick
- 1 Granny Smith apple, not peeled, cored and cut into ½-inch wedges

Directions:

1. Preheat the toaster oven to 375°F. Spray a 12 x 12-inch baking pan with nonstick cooking spray.

2. Place the sweet potatoes on one side of the prepared pan. Spray with nonstick cooking spray. Bake, uncovered, for 20 minutes.

3. Meanwhile, stir the bourbon, honey, oil, onion powder, mustard, and thyme in a small bowl. Season with salt and pepper and set aside.

4. Turn the potatoes over. Place the pork chops on the other end of the pan in a single layer. Arrange the apple wedges around the potatoes and pork chops, stacking the apples as needed. Brush the bourbon mixture generously over all. Bake for 15 to 18 minutes or until the pork is done as desired and a meat thermometer registers a minimum of 145°F.

5. For additional browning, set the toaster oven to Broil and broil for 2 to 4 minutes, or until the edges are brown as desired.

6. Transfer to a serving platter. Spoon any drippings over the meat and vegetables. Let stand for 5 minutes before serving.

SNACKS APPETIZERS AND SIDES

Corn Dog Muffins

Servings: 8
Cooking Time: 10 Minutes

Ingredients:

- 1¼ cups sliced kosher hotdogs (3 or 4, depending on size)
- ½ cup flour
- ½ cup yellow cornmeal
- 2 teaspoons baking powder
- ½ cup skim milk
- 1 egg
- 2 tablespoons canola oil
- 8 foil muffin cups, paper liners removed
- cooking spray
- mustard or your favorite dipping sauce

Directions:

1. Slice each hot dog in half lengthwise, then cut in ¼-inch half-moon slices. Set aside.
2. Preheat the toaster oven to 390°F.
3. In a large bowl, stir together flour, cornmeal, and baking powder.
4. In a small bowl, beat together the milk, egg, and oil until just blended.
5. Pour egg mixture into dry ingredients and stir with a spoon to mix well.
6. Stir in sliced hot dogs.
7. Spray the foil cups lightly with cooking spray.
8. Divide mixture evenly into muffin cups.
9. Place 4 muffin cups in the air fryer oven and air-fry for 5 minutes.
10. Reduce temperature to 360°F and cook 5 minutes or until toothpick inserted in center of muffin comes out clean.
11. Repeat steps 9 and 10 to bake remaining corn dog muffins.
12. Serve with mustard or other sauces for dipping.

Sugar-glazed Walnuts

Servings: 6
Cooking Time: 5 Minutes

Ingredients:

- 1 Large egg white(s)
- 2 tablespoons Granulated white sugar
- ⅛ teaspoon Table salt
- 2 cups (7 ounces) Walnut halves

Directions:

1. Preheat the toaster oven to 400°F.
2. Use a whisk to beat the egg white(s) in a large bowl until quite foamy, more so than just well combined but certainly not yet a meringue.
3. If you're working with the quantities for a small batch, remove half of the foamy egg white.
4. If you're working with the quantities for a large batch, remove a quarter of it. It's fine to eyeball the amounts.
5. You can store the removed egg white in a sealed container to save for another use.
6. Stir in the sugar and salt. Add the walnut halves and toss to coat evenly and well, including the nuts' crevasses.
7. When the machine is at temperature, use a slotted spoon to transfer the walnut halves to the air fryer oven, taking care not to dislodge any coating. Gently spread the nuts into as close to one layer as you can. Air-fry undisturbed for 2 minutes.
8. Break up any clumps, toss the walnuts gently but well, and air-fry for 3 minutes more, tossing after 1 minute, then every 30 seconds thereafter,

until the nuts are browned in spots and very aromatic. Watch carefully so they don't burn.

9. Gently dump the nuts onto a lipped baking sheet and spread them into one layer. Cool for at least 10 minutes before serving, separating any that stick together. The walnuts can be stored in a sealed container at room temperature for up to 5 days.

Bacon Corn Muffins

Servings: 6
Cooking Time: 17 Minutes

Ingredients:

- 1 1/4 cups self rising cornmeal mix
- 3/4 cup buttermilk
- 1/3 cup chopped cooked bacon
- 1/4 cup butter, melted
- 1 large egg, slightly beaten

Directions:

1. Preheat toaster oven to 425°F on CONVECTION setting.
2. Stir cornmeal mix, buttermilk, bacon, butter and egg until blended.
3. Spoon batter into lightly greased muffin pan, filling 3/4 full.
4. Bake 15 to 17 minutes until toothpick inserted in center comes out clean.
5. Cool 10 minutes on wire rack; remove.

Creamy Crab Dip

Servings: 4
Cooking Time: 20 Minutes

Ingredients:

- 6 ounces cream cheese, room temperature
- ½ cup sour cream
- ½ cup grated Parmesan cheese
- ½ cup shredded cheddar cheese
- Juice of ½ lemon

- ½ teaspoon garlic powder
- Dash hot sauce
- 1 (6-ounce) can crab meat, drained
- Sea salt, for seasoning
- Freshly ground black pepper, for seasoning
- Baguette, cut into ¼-inch-wide rounds, for serving

Directions:

1. Place the rack on position 1 and preheat the toaster oven on BAKE to 400°F for 5 minutes.
2. In a medium bowl, stir the cream cheese, sour cream, Parmesan, cheddar, lemon juice, garlic powder, and hot sauce until well blended.
3. Fold in the crab and season with salt and pepper.
4. Spoon the dip into a shallow heatproof 4-cup bowl.
5. Bake for 20 minutes until golden and bubbling.
6. Serve with baguette slices.

Sesame Green Beans

Servings: 4
Cooking Time: 8 Minutes

Ingredients:

- 1 pound green beans, stems trimmed
- 1 tablespoon olive oil
- 1 teaspoon sesame oil
- 1 tablespoon sesame seeds
- Pinch sea salt

Directions:

1. Preheat the toaster oven to 350°F on AIR FRY for 5 minutes.
2. In a large bowl, toss the green beans, olive oil, and sesame oil.
3. Place the air-fryer basket in the baking tray and spread the beans in the basket.

4. Place the tray in position 2 and air fry for 8 minutes, shaking the basket at the halfway point. The beans should be lightly golden and fragrant.

5. Transfer the beans to a serving plate and serve topped with the sesame seeds and seasoned with salt.

Crab Rangoon Dip With Wonton Chips

Servings: 6
Cooking Time: 18 Minutes

Ingredients:

- Wonton Chips:
- 1 (12-ounce) package wonton wrappers
- vegetable oil
- sea salt
- Crab Rangoon Dip:
- 8 ounces cream cheese, softened
- ¾ cup sour cream
- 1 teaspoon Worcestershire sauce
- 1½ teaspoons soy sauce
- 1 teaspoon sesame oil
- ⅛ teaspoon ground cayenne pepper
- ¼ teaspoon salt
- freshly ground black pepper
- 8 ounces cooked crabmeat
- 1 cup grated white Cheddar cheese
- ⅓ cup chopped scallions
- paprika (for garnish)

Directions:

1. Cut the wonton wrappers in half diagonally to form triangles. Working in batches, lay the wonton triangles on a flat surface and brush or spray both sides with vegetable oil.

2. Preheat the toaster oven to 370°F.

3. Place about 10 to 12 wonton triangles in the air fryer oven, letting them overlap slightly. Air-fry for just 2 minutes. Transfer the wonton chips to a large bowl and season immediately with sea salt. (You'll hear the chips start to spin around in the air fryer oven when they are almost done.) Repeat with the rest of wontons (keeping those fishing hands at bay!).

4. To make the dip, combine the cream cheese, sour cream, Worcestershire sauce, soy sauce, sesame oil, cayenne pepper, salt, and freshly ground black pepper in a bowl. Mix well and then fold in the crabmeat, Cheddar cheese, and scallions.

5. Transfer the dip to a 7-inch ceramic baking pan or shallow casserole dish. Sprinkle paprika on top and cover the dish with aluminum foil. Lower the dish into the air fryer oven using a sling made of aluminum foil (fold a piece of aluminum foil into a strip about 2-inches wide by 24-inches long). Air-fry for 11 minutes. Remove the aluminum foil and air-fry for another 5 minutes to finish cooking and brown the top. Serve hot with the wonton chips.

Roasted Green Beans With Goat Cheese And Hazelnuts

Servings: 2
Cooking Time: 45 Minutes

Ingredients:

- 12 ounces green beans, trimmed
- 3 tablespoons extra-virgin olive oil, divided
- ¼ teaspoon sugar
- ¼ teaspoon plus ⅛ teaspoon table salt, divided
- ¼ teaspoon plus ⅛ teaspoon pepper, divided
- 1 garlic clove, minced
- ½ teaspoon grated orange zest plus 1 teaspoon juice
- 1 teaspoon lemon juice
- ½ teaspoon Dijon mustard
- 1 tablespoon minced fresh chives

- 1 ounce goat cheese, crumbled (¼ cup)
- 2 tablespoons chopped toasted hazelnuts

Directions:

1. Adjust toaster oven rack to lowest position and preheat the toaster oven to 450 degrees. Toss green beans, 1 tablespoon oil, sugar, ¼ teaspoon salt, and ¼ teaspoon pepper together in bowl, then spread into even layer on small rimmed baking sheet.

2. Cover sheet tightly with aluminum foil and roast for 12 minutes. Remove foil and continue to roast until green beans are spotty brown, 10 to 15 minutes.

3. Meanwhile, combine garlic, orange zest, and remaining 2 tablespoons oil in large bowl and microwave until fragrant, 30 to 60 seconds; let steep for 1 minute. Whisk in orange juice, lemon juice, mustard, remaining ⅛ teaspoon salt, and remaining ⅛ teaspoon pepper. Add green beans and chives and toss to combine. Transfer to serving platter and sprinkle with goat cheese and hazelnuts. Serve.

Simple Holiday Stuffing

Servings: 4
Cooking Time: 120 Minutes

Ingredients:

- 12 ounces hearty white sandwich bread, cut into ½-inch pieces (8 cups)
- 1 onion, chopped fine
- 1 celery rib, chopped fine
- 1 tablespoon unsalted butter, plus 5 tablespoons, melted
- 1 tablespoon minced fresh thyme or 1 teaspoon dried
- 2 teaspoons minced fresh sage or ½ teaspoon dried
- ¾ teaspoon table salt

- ¼ teaspoon pepper
- 1¼ cups chicken broth

Directions:

1. Adjust toaster oven rack to middle position and preheat the toaster oven to 300 degrees. Spread bread into even layer on small rimmed baking sheet and bake until light golden brown, 35 to 45 minutes, tossing halfway through baking. Let bread cool completely on sheet.

2. Increase oven temperature to 375 degrees. Microwave onion, celery, 1 tablespoon butter, thyme, sage, salt, and pepper in covered large bowl, stirring occasionally, until vegetables are softened, 2 to 4 minutes.

3. Stir in broth, then add bread and toss to combine. Let mixture sit for 10 minutes, then toss mixture again until broth is fully absorbed. Transfer bread mixture to 8-inch square baking dish or pan and distribute evenly but do not pack down. (Stuffing can be covered and refrigerated for up to 24 hours; increase covered baking time to 15 minutes.)

4. Drizzle melted butter evenly over top of stuffing. Cover dish tightly with aluminum foil and bake for 10 minutes. Uncover and continue to bake until top is golden brown and crisp, 15 to 25 minutes. Transfer dish to wire rack and let cool for 10 minutes. Serve.

Baked Brie And Cranberry Bites

Servings: 24
Cooking Time: 10 Minutes

Ingredients:

- 4 ounces triple creme brie
- 1/4 cup Cranberry Orange Relish
- 4 sheets phyllo pastry sheets, thawed
- 1/4 cup butter, melted

Directions:

1. Preheat the toaster oven to 400°F.

2. Cut brie into 1/4-inch slices, then in 1-inch pieces; set aside.

3. Unroll and cover the phyllo sheets with plastic wrap and then a slightly damp towel to prevent drying out. On a large cutting board, place one sheet of phyllo. Lightly brush with melted butter. Continue to layer phyllo sheets and brush with butter, but do not butter the top of the last sheet.

4. Cut the layered phyllo sheets into 24 equal squares. Place each square in a mini-muffin pan, pushing down center to form a cup. Keep cut squares and already shaped phyllo cups covered with plastic wrap and a damp towel to prevent drying out while shaping more squares.

5. Place a piece of brie in each phyllo cup in muffin pans. Top with 1/2 teaspoon cranberry relish.

6. Bake 8 to 10 minutes or until golden brown.

Garlic Parmesan Kale Chips

Servings: 2

Cooking Time: 6 Minutes

Ingredients:

- 16 large kale leaves, washed and thick stems removed
- 1 tablespoon avocado oil
- ½ teaspoon garlic powder
- 1 teaspoon soy sauce or tamari
- ¼ cup grated Parmesan cheese

Directions:

1. Preheat the toaster oven to 370°F.

2. Make a stack of kale leaves and cut them into 4 pieces.

3. Place the kale pieces into a large bowl. Drizzle the avocado oil onto the kale and rub to coat. Add the garlic powder, soy sauce or tamari, and cheese, tossing to coat.

4. Pour the chips into the air fryer oven and air-fry for 6 minutes, checking for crispness every minute. When done cooking, pour the kale chips onto paper towels and cool at least 5 minutes before serving.

Savory Sausage Balls

Servings: 10

Cooking Time: 8 Minutes

Ingredients:

- 2 cups all-purpose flour
- 1 tablespoon baking powder
- ½ teaspoon garlic powder
- ¼ teaspoon onion powder
- ½ teaspoon salt
- 3 tablespoons milk
- 2½ cups grated pepper jack cheese
- 1 pound fresh sausage, casing removed

Directions:

1. Preheat the toaster oven to 370°F.

2. In a large bowl, whisk together the flour, baking powder, garlic powder, onion powder, and salt. Add in the milk, grated cheese, and sausage.

3. Using a tablespoon, scoop out the sausage and roll it between your hands to form a rounded ball. You should end up with approximately 32 balls. Place them in the air fryer oven in a single layer and working in batches as necessary.

4. Air-fry for 8 minutes, or until the outer coating turns light brown.

5. Carefully remove, repeating with the remaining sausage balls.

Rosemary-roasted Potatoes

Servings:4
Cooking Time: 40 Minutes

Ingredients:
- 1 pound russet potatoes, or baby potatoes, cut into 1-inch chunks
- 2 tablespoons olive oil
- 1 teaspoon garlic powder
- 1 teaspoon dried rosemary
- Sea salt, for seasoning
- Freshly ground black pepper, for seasoning

Directions:
1. Preheat the toaster oven on AIR FRY to 400°F for 5 minutes.
2. In a large bowl, toss the potatoes with the oil, garlic powder, and rosemary. Season with salt and pepper.
3. Place the air-fryer basket in the baking tray and spread the potatoes in a single layer in the basket. You may have to do two batches. Cover the first batch loosely with foil to keep it warm while you cook the second batch.
4. In position 2, AIR FRY on 400°F for 20 minutes, shaking the basket at 10 minutes, until the potatoes are tender and golden brown. Repeat with the remaining potatoes and serve.

Sweet Potato Casserole

Servings: 4
Cooking Time: 90 Minutes

Ingredients:
- 2 tablespoons packed brown sugar, divided
- ½ teaspoon grated orange zest, divided, plus 1 tablespoon juice
- 1½ pounds sweet potatoes, peeled and cut into 1½-inch pieces
- 2 tablespoons unsalted butter, cut into 4 pieces

- 2 tablespoons heavy cream
- ½ teaspoon table salt
- ¼ teaspoon ground cinnamon
- ⅛ teaspoon pepper
- Pinch cayenne pepper

Directions:
1. Adjust toaster oven rack to middle position and preheat the toaster oven to 400 degrees. Mix 4 teaspoons sugar and ¼ teaspoon orange zest in small bowl until thoroughly combined; set aside.
2. Toss sweet potatoes and remaining 2 teaspoons sugar together in bowl, then spread into even layer on aluminum foil–lined small rimmed baking sheet. Cover sheet tightly with foil and roast until sweet potatoes are tender, 45 to 60 minutes, rotating sheet halfway through roasting. Remove sheet from oven, select broiler function, and heat broiler.
3. Transfer potatoes and any accumulated liquid to food processor. Add butter, cream, salt, cinnamon, pepper, cayenne, remaining ¼ teaspoon orange zest, and orange juice and process until completely smooth, 30 to 60 seconds, scraping down sides of bowl as needed.
4. Transfer potato puree to 8-inch square broiler-safe baking dish or pan and sprinkle evenly with reserved sugar-zest mixture. Broil sweet potatoes until topping is melted and beginning to caramelize, 10 to 12 minutes. Transfer dish to wire rack and let cool for 10 minutes. Serve.

Blistered Shishito Peppers

Servings: 3
Cooking Time: 5 Minutes

Ingredients:
- 6 ounces (about 18) Shishito peppers
- Vegetable oil spray

- For garnishing Coarse sea or kosher salt and lemon wedges

Directions:

1. Preheat the toaster oven to 400°F.

2. Put the peppers in a bowl and lightly coat them with vegetable oil spray. Toss gently, spray again, and toss until the peppers are glistening but not drenched.

3. Pour the peppers into the pan, spread them into as close to one layer as you can, and air-fry for 5 minutes, tossing and rearranging the peppers at the 2- and 4-minute marks, until the peppers are blistered and even blackened in spots.

4. Pour the peppers into a bowl, add salt to taste, and toss gently. Serve the peppers with lemon wedges to squeeze over them.

Garlic Breadsticks

Servings: 12
Cooking Time: 7 Minutes

Ingredients:
- 1½ tablespoons Olive oil
- 1½ teaspoons Minced garlic
- ¼ teaspoon Table salt
- ¼ teaspoon Ground black pepper
- 6 ounces Purchased pizza dough (vegan dough, if that's a concern)

Directions:

1. Preheat the toaster oven to 400°F. Mix the oil, garlic, salt, and pepper in a small bowl.

2. Divide the pizza dough into 4 balls for a small air fryer oven, 6 for a medium machine, or 8 for a large, each ball about the size of a walnut in its shell. (Each should weigh 1 ounce, if you want to drag out a scale and get obsessive.) Roll each ball into a 5-inch-long stick under your clean palms on a clean, dry work surface. Brush the sticks with the oil mixture.

3. When the machine is at temperature, place the prepared dough sticks in the air fryer oven, leaving a 1-inch space between them. Air-fry undisturbed for 7 minutes, or until puffed, golden, and set to the touch.

4. Use kitchen tongs to gently transfer the breadsticks to a wire rack and repeat step 3 with the remaining dough sticks.

Parmesan Garlic French Fries

Servings: 4
Cooking Time: 25 Minutes

Ingredients:
- 16 ounces frozen regular-cut french fries
- 2 tablespoons olive oil
- 1 teaspoon Italian seasoning
- ½ teaspoon garlic powder
- ½ teaspoon kosher salt
- ¼ teaspoon freshly ground black pepper
- ¼ cup grated Parmesan cheese
- 2 tablespoons minced fresh flat-leaf (Italian) parsley

Directions:

1. Preheat the toaster oven to 425°F. Line a 12 x 12-inch baking pan with nonstick aluminum foil (or if lining the pan with regular foil, spray it with nonstick cooking spray).

2. Place the french fries in a large bowl. Drizzle with the olive oil and toss to coat the fries evenly.

3. Blend the Italian seasoning, garlic powder, salt, and pepper in a small bowl. Sprinkle the seasonings over the fries and toss to coat evenly. Spread the fries in a single layer in the prepared pan.

4. Bake, uncovered, for 10 minutes. Stir and bake for an additional 10 to 15 minutes, or until the fries are golden brown and crisp.

5. Remove the fries from the oven and immediately sprinkle with the Parmesan cheese and parsley. Toss gently to coat them evenly.

- ¼ cup canned artichoke hearts, drained and patted dry
- ¼ cup frozen spinach, defrosted and squeezed dry
- 2 ounces cream cheese
- 1½ teaspoons dried oregano, divided
- ¼ teaspoon garlic powder
- ¼ teaspoon onion powder
- ½ teaspoon salt
- ¼ cup chopped pepperoni
- ¼ cup grated mozzarella cheese
- 1 tablespoon grated Parmesan
- 2 ounces cream cheese
- ½ teaspoon dried oregano
- 32 wontons
- 1 cup water

Directions:

1. Preheat the toaster oven to 370°F.
2. In a medium bowl, mix together the refried beans and salsa.
3. In a second medium bowl, mix together the artichoke hearts, spinach, cream cheese, oregano, garlic powder, onion powder, and salt.
4. In a third medium bowl, mix together the pepperoni, mozzarella cheese, Parmesan cheese, cream cheese, and the remaining ½ teaspoon of oregano.
5. Get a towel lightly damp with water and ring it out. While working with the wontons, leave the unfilled wontons under the damp towel so they don't dry out.
6. Working with 8 wontons at a time, place 2 teaspoons of one of the fillings into the center of the wonton, rotating among the different fillings (one filling per wonton). Working one at a time, use a pastry brush, dip the pastry brush into the water, and brush the edges of the dough with the water. Fold the dough in half to form a triangle

and set aside. Continue until 8 wontons are formed. Spray the wontons with cooking spray and cover with a dry towel. Repeat until all 32 wontons have been filled.
7. Place the wontons into the air fryer oven, leaving space between the wontons, and air-fry for 5 minutes. Turn over and check for brownness, and then air-fry for another 5 minutes.

Cherry Chipotle Bbq Chicken Wings

Servings: 2
Cooking Time: 12 Minutes

Ingredients:

- 1 teaspoon smoked paprika
- ½ teaspoon dry mustard powder
- 1 teaspoon dried oregano
- 1 teaspoon dried thyme
- ½ teaspoon chili powder
- 1 teaspoon salt
- 2 pounds chicken wings
- vegetable oil or spray
- salt and freshly ground black pepper
- 1 to 2 tablespoons chopped chipotle peppers in adobo sauce
- ⅓ cup cherry preserves ¼ cup tomato ketchup

Directions:

1. Combine the first six ingredients in a large bowl. Prepare the chicken wings by cutting off the wing tips and discarding (or freezing for chicken stock). Divide the drumettes from the win-gettes by cutting through the joint. Place the chicken wing pieces in the bowl with the spice mix. Toss or shake well to coat.
2. Preheat the toaster oven to 400°F.
3. Spray the wings lightly with the vegetable oil and air-fry the wings in two batches for 10 minutes per batch. When both batches are done, toss all the wings back into the air fryer oven for

Granola Three Ways

Servings: 4
Cooking Time: 10 Minutes

Ingredients:

- Nantucket Granola
- ¼ cup maple syrup
- ¼ cup dark brown sugar
- 1 tablespoon butter
- 1 teaspoon vanilla extract
- 1 cup rolled oats
- ½ cup dried cranberries
- ½ cup walnuts, chopped
- ¼ cup pumpkin seeds
- ¼ cup shredded coconut
- Blueberry Delight
- ¼ cup honey
- ¼ cup light brown sugar
- 1 tablespoon butter
- 1 teaspoon lemon extract
- 1 cup rolled oats
- ½ cup sliced almonds
- ½ cup dried blueberries
- ¼ cup pumpkin seeds
- ¼ cup sunflower seeds
- Cherry Black Forest Mix
- ¼ cup honey
- ¼ cup light brown sugar
- 1 tablespoon butter
- 1 teaspoon almond extract
- 1 cup rolled oats
- ½ cup sliced almonds
- ½ cup dried cherries
- ¼ cup shredded coconut
- ¼ cup dark chocolate chips
- oil for misting or cooking spray

Directions:

1. Combine the syrup or honey, brown sugar, and butter in a small saucepan or microwave-safe bowl. Heat and stir just until butter melts and sugar dissolves. Stir in the extract.
2. Place all other dry ingredients in a large bowl. (For the Cherry Black Forest Mix, don't add the chocolate chips yet.)
3. Pour melted butter mixture over dry ingredients and stir until oat mixture is well coated.
4. Lightly spray a baking pan with oil or cooking spray.
5. Pour granola into pan and air-fry at 390°F for 5 minutes. Stir. Continue cooking for 5 minutes, stirring every minute or two, until golden brown. Watch closely. Once the mixture begins to brown, it will cook quickly.
6. Remove granola from pan and spread on wax paper. It will become crispier as it cools.
7. For the Cherry Black Forest Mix, stir in chocolate chips after granola has cooled completely.
8. Store in an airtight container.

Veggie Cheese Bites

Servings: 4
Cooking Time: 8 Minutes

Ingredients:

- 2 cups riced vegetables
- ½ cup shredded zucchini
- ½ teaspoon garlic powder
- ¼ teaspoon black pepper
- ¼ teaspoon salt
- 1 large egg
- ¾ cup shredded cheddar cheese
- ⅓ cup whole-wheat flour

Directions:

1. Preheat the toaster oven to 350°F.

2. In a large bowl, mix together the riced vegetables, zucchini, garlic powder, pepper, and salt. Mix in the egg. Stir in the shredded cheese and whole-wheat flour until a thick, doughlike consistency forms. If you need to, add 1 teaspoon of flour at a time so you can mold the batter into balls.

3. Using a 1-inch scoop, portion the batter out into about 12 balls.

4. Liberally spray the air fryer oven with olive oil spray. Then place the veggie bites inside. Leave enough room between each bite so the air can flow around them.

5. Air-fry for 8 minutes, or until the outside is slightly browned. Depending on the size of your air fryer oven, you may need to cook these in batches.

6. Remove and let cool slightly before serving.

Loaded Potato Skins

Servings: 8
Cooking Time: 8 Minutes

Ingredients:

- 12 round baby potatoes
- 3 ounces cream cheese
- 4 slices cooked bacon, crumbled or chopped
- 2 green onions, finely chopped
- ½ cup grated cheddar cheese, divided
- ¼ cup sour cream
- 1 tablespoon milk
- 2 teaspoons hot sauce

Directions:

1. Preheat the toaster oven to 320°F.

2. Poke holes into the baby potatoes with a fork. Place the potatoes onto a microwave-safe plate and microwave on high for 4 to 5 minutes, or until soft to squeeze. Let the potatoes cool until they're safe to handle, about 5 minutes.

3. Meanwhile, in a medium bowl, mix together the cream cheese, bacon, green onions, and ¼ cup of the cheddar cheese; set aside.

4. Slice the baby potatoes in half. Using a spoon, scoop out the pulp, leaving enough pulp on the inside to retain the shape of the potato half. Place the potato pulp into the cream cheese mixture and mash together with a fork. Using a spoon, refill the potato halves with filling.

5. Place the potato halves into the air fryer oven and top with the remaining ¼ cup of cheddar cheese.

6. Cook the loaded baked potato bites in batches for 8 minutes.

7. Meanwhile, make the sour cream sauce. In a small bowl, whisk together the sour cream, milk, and hot sauce. Add more hot sauce if desired.

8. When the potatoes have all finished cooking, place them onto a serving platter and serve with sour cream sauce drizzled over the top or as a dip.

Roasted Pumpkin Seeds

Servings: 2-4
Cooking Time: 50 Minutes

Ingredients:

- 1 medium pumpkin
- 1 tablespoon vegetable oil
- Salt

Directions:

1. Preheat the toaster oven to 300°F. Line a baking sheet with parchment paper. Set aside.

2. Cut the top from the pumpkin. Using a large spoon, scrape out the pulp and seeds from the pumpkin and place in a colander or strainer.

3. Separate the pulp and strings from seeds. Rinse seeds and pat dry with paper towels.

4. Spread the seeds on the prepared baking sheet.

5. Bake until the seeds are dry, about 30 minutes.

6. In a small bowl, toss seeds with oil and salt. Bake until seeds are toasted, an additional 15 to 20 minutes.

Baba Ghanouj

Servings: 2
Cooking Time: 40 Minutes

Ingredients:

- 2 Small (12-ounce) purple Italian eggplant(s)
- ¼ cup Olive oil
- ¼ cup Tahini
- ½ teaspoon Ground black pepper
- ¼ teaspoon Onion powder
- ¼ teaspoon Mild smoked paprika (optional)
- Up to 1 teaspoon Table salt

Directions:

1. Preheat the toaster oven to 400°F.

2. Prick the eggplant(s) on all sides with a fork. When the machine is at temperature, set the eggplant(s) in the air fryer oven in one layer. Air-fry undisturbed for 40 minutes, or until blackened and soft.

3. Remove from the machine. Cool the eggplant(s) in the air fryer oven for 20 minutes.

4. Use a nonstick-safe spatula, and perhaps a flatware tablespoon for balance, to gently transfer the eggplant(s) to a bowl. The juices will run out. Make sure the bowl is close to the air fryer oven. Split the eggplant(s) open.

5. Scrape the soft insides of half an eggplant into a food processor. Repeat with the remaining piece(s). Add any juices from the bowl to the eggplant in the food processor, but discard the skins and stems.

6. Add the olive oil, tahini, pepper, onion powder, and smoked paprika (if using). Add about half the salt, then cover and process until smooth, stopping the machine at least once to scrape down the inside of the canister. Check the spread for salt and add more as needed. Scrape the baba ghanouj into a bowl and serve warm, or

set aside at room temperature for up to or cover and store in the refrigerator for days.

Brazilian Cheese Bread (pão Queijo)

Servings: 8
Cooking Time: 18 Minutes

Ingredients:

- 1 large egg, room temperature
- ⅓ cup olive oil
- ⅔ cups whole milk 1½ cups tapioca flour
- ½ cup feta cheese
- ¼ cup Parmesan cheese
- 1 teaspoon kosher salt
- ¼ teaspoon garlic powder
- Cooking spray

Directions:

1. Blend the egg, olive oil, milk, tapioca fl feta, Parmesan, salt, and garlic powder in a s mixer until smooth.

2. Spray the mini muffin pan with cooking s

3. Pour the batter into the muffin cups so are ¾ full.

4. .Preheat the toaster oven to 380°F.

5. Place the muffin pan on the wire rack, insert rack at mid position in the preheated ov

6. Select the Bake function, adjust time to minutes, and press Start/Pause.

7. Remove when done, then carefully pop bread from the mini muffin tin and serve.

Crispy Wontons

Servings: 8
Cooking Time: 10 Minutes

Ingredients:

- ½ cup refried beans
- 3 tablespoons salsa

Granola Three Ways

Servings: 4

Cooking Time: 10 Minutes

Ingredients:

- Nantucket Granola
- ¼ cup maple syrup
- ¼ cup dark brown sugar
- 1 tablespoon butter
- 1 teaspoon vanilla extract
- 1 cup rolled oats
- ½ cup dried cranberries
- ½ cup walnuts, chopped
- ¼ cup pumpkin seeds
- ¼ cup shredded coconut
- Blueberry Delight
- ¼ cup honey
- ¼ cup light brown sugar
- 1 tablespoon butter
- 1 teaspoon lemon extract
- 1 cup rolled oats
- ½ cup sliced almonds
- ½ cup dried blueberries
- ¼ cup pumpkin seeds
- ¼ cup sunflower seeds
- Cherry Black Forest Mix
- ¼ cup honey
- ¼ cup light brown sugar
- 1 tablespoon butter
- 1 teaspoon almond extract
- 1 cup rolled oats
- ½ cup sliced almonds
- ½ cup dried cherries
- ¼ cup shredded coconut
- ¼ cup dark chocolate chips
- oil for misting or cooking spray

Directions:

1. Combine the syrup or honey, brown sugar, and butter in a small saucepan or microwave-safe bowl. Heat and stir just until butter melts and sugar dissolves. Stir in the extract.

2. Place all other dry ingredients in a large bowl. (For the Cherry Black Forest Mix, don't add the chocolate chips yet.)

3. Pour melted butter mixture over dry ingredients and stir until oat mixture is well coated.

4. Lightly spray a baking pan with oil or cooking spray.

5. Pour granola into pan and air-fry at 390°F for 5 minutes. Stir. Continue cooking for 5 minutes, stirring every minute or two, until golden brown. Watch closely. Once the mixture begins to brown, it will cook quickly.

6. Remove granola from pan and spread on wax paper. It will become crispier as it cools.

7. For the Cherry Black Forest Mix, stir in chocolate chips after granola has cooled completely.

8. Store in an airtight container.

Veggie Cheese Bites

Servings: 4

Cooking Time: 8 Minutes

Ingredients:

- 2 cups riced vegetables
- ½ cup shredded zucchini
- ½ teaspoon garlic powder
- ¼ teaspoon black pepper
- ¼ teaspoon salt
- 1 large egg
- ¾ cup shredded cheddar cheese
- ⅓ cup whole-wheat flour

Directions:

1. Preheat the toaster oven to 350°F.

2. In a large bowl, mix together the riced vegetables, zucchini, garlic powder, pepper, and salt. Mix in the egg. Stir in the shredded cheese and whole-wheat flour until a thick, doughlike consistency forms. If you need to, add 1 teaspoon of flour at a time so you can mold the batter into balls.

3. Using a 1-inch scoop, portion the batter out into about 12 balls.

4. Liberally spray the air fryer oven with olive oil spray. Then place the veggie bites inside. Leave enough room between each bite so the air can flow around them.

5. Air-fry for 8 minutes, or until the outside is slightly browned. Depending on the size of your air fryer oven, you may need to cook these in batches.

6. Remove and let cool slightly before serving.

Loaded Potato Skins

Servings: 8
Cooking Time: 8 Minutes

Ingredients:
- 12 round baby potatoes
- 3 ounces cream cheese
- 4 slices cooked bacon, crumbled or chopped
- 2 green onions, finely chopped
- ½ cup grated cheddar cheese, divided
- ¼ cup sour cream
- 1 tablespoon milk
- 2 teaspoons hot sauce

Directions:
1. Preheat the toaster oven to 320°F.

2. Poke holes into the baby potatoes with a fork. Place the potatoes onto a microwave-safe plate and microwave on high for 4 to 5 minutes, or until soft to squeeze. Let the potatoes cool until they're safe to handle, about 5 minutes.

3. Meanwhile, in a medium bowl, mix together the cream cheese, bacon, green onions, and ¼ cup of the cheddar cheese; set aside.

4. Slice the baby potatoes in half. Using a spoon, scoop out the pulp, leaving enough pulp on the inside to retain the shape of the potato half. Place the potato pulp into the cream cheese mixture and mash together with a fork. Using a spoon, refill the potato halves with filling.

5. Place the potato halves into the air fryer oven and top with the remaining ¼ cup of cheddar cheese.

6. Cook the loaded baked potato bites in batches for 8 minutes.

7. Meanwhile, make the sour cream sauce. In a small bowl, whisk together the sour cream, milk, and hot sauce. Add more hot sauce if desired.

8. When the potatoes have all finished cooking, place them onto a serving platter and serve with sour cream sauce drizzled over the top or as a dip.

Roasted Pumpkin Seeds

Servings: 2-4
Cooking Time: 50 Minutes

Ingredients:
- 1 medium pumpkin
- 1 tablespoon vegetable oil
- Salt

Directions:
1. Preheat the toaster oven to 300°F. Line a baking sheet with parchment paper. Set aside.

2. Cut the top from the pumpkin. Using a large spoon, scrape out the pulp and seeds from the pumpkin and place in a colander or strainer.

3. Separate the pulp and strings from seeds. Rinse seeds and pat dry with paper towels.

4. Spread the seeds on the prepared baking sheet.

5. Bake until the seeds are dry, about 30 minutes.

6. In a small bowl, toss seeds with oil and salt. Bake until seeds are toasted, an additional 15 to 20 minutes.

Baba Ghanouj

Servings: 2

Cooking Time: 40 Minutes

Ingredients:

- 2 Small (12-ounce) purple Italian eggplant(s)
- ¼ cup Olive oil
- ¼ cup Tahini
- ½ teaspoon Ground black pepper
- ¼ teaspoon Onion powder
- ¼ teaspoon Mild smoked paprika (optional)
- Up to 1 teaspoon Table salt

Directions:

1. Preheat the toaster oven to 400°F.

2. Prick the eggplant(s) on all sides with a fork. When the machine is at temperature, set the eggplant(s) in the air fryer oven in one layer. Air-fry undisturbed for 40 minutes, or until blackened and soft.

3. Remove from the machine. Cool the eggplant(s) in the air fryer oven for 20 minutes.

4. Use a nonstick-safe spatula, and perhaps a flatware tablespoon for balance, to gently transfer the eggplant(s) to a bowl. The juices will run out. Make sure the bowl is close to the air fryer oven. Split the eggplant(s) open.

5. Scrape the soft insides of half an eggplant into a food processor. Repeat with the remaining piece(s). Add any juices from the bowl to the eggplant in the food processor, but discard the skins and stems.

6. Add the olive oil, tahini, pepper, onion powder, and smoked paprika (if using). Add about half the salt, then cover and process until smooth, stopping the machine at least once to scrape down the inside of the canister. Check the spread for salt and add more as needed. Scrape the baba ghanouj into a bowl and serve warm, or

set aside at room temperature for up to 2 hours, or cover and store in the refrigerator for up to 4 days.

Brazilian Cheese Bread (pão De Queijo)

Servings: 8

Cooking Time: 18 Minutes

Ingredients:

- 1 large egg, room temperature
- ⅓ cup olive oil
- ⅔ cups whole milk 1½ cups tapioca flour
- ½ cup feta cheese
- ¼ cup Parmesan cheese
- 1 teaspoon kosher salt
- ¼ teaspoon garlic powder
- Cooking spray

Directions:

1. Blend the egg, olive oil, milk, tapioca flour, feta, Parmesan, salt, and garlic powder in a stand mixer until smooth.

2. Spray the mini muffin pan with cooking spray.

3. Pour the batter into the muffin cups so they are ¾ full.

4. .Preheat the toaster oven to 380°F.

5. Place the muffin pan on the wire rack, then insert rack at mid position in the preheated oven.

6. Select the Bake function, adjust time to 18 minutes, and press Start/Pause.

7. Remove when done, then carefully pop the bread from the mini muffin tin and serve.

Crispy Wontons

Servings: 8

Cooking Time: 10 Minutes

Ingredients:

- ½ cup refried beans
- 3 tablespoons salsa

- ¼ cup canned artichoke hearts, drained and patted dry
- ¼ cup frozen spinach, defrosted and squeezed dry
- 2 ounces cream cheese
- 1½ teaspoons dried oregano, divided
- ¼ teaspoon garlic powder
- ¼ teaspoon onion powder
- ½ teaspoon salt
- ¼ cup chopped pepperoni
- ¼ cup grated mozzarella cheese
- 1 tablespoon grated Parmesan
- 2 ounces cream cheese
- ½ teaspoon dried oregano
- 32 wontons
- 1 cup water

Directions:

1. Preheat the toaster oven to 370°F.

2. In a medium bowl, mix together the refried beans and salsa.

3. In a second medium bowl, mix together the_ artichoke hearts, spinach, cream cheese, oregano, garlic powder, onion powder, and salt.

4. In a third medium bowl, mix together the pepperoni, mozzarella cheese, Parmesan cheese, cream cheese, and the remaining ½ teaspoon of oregano.

5. Get a towel lightly damp with water and ring it out. While working with the wontons, leave the unfilled wontons under the damp towel so they don't dry out.

6. Working with 8 wontons at a time, place 2 teaspoons of one of the fillings into the center of the wonton, rotating among the different fillings (one filling per wonton). Working one at a time, use a pastry brush, dip the pastry brush into the water, and brush the edges of the dough with the water. Fold the dough in half to form a triangle

and set aside. Continue until 8 wontons are formed. Spray the wontons with cooking spray and cover with a dry towel. Repeat until all 32 wontons have been filled.

7. Place the wontons into the air fryer oven, leaving space between the wontons, and air-fry for 5 minutes. Turn over and check for brownness, and then air-fry for another 5 minutes.

Cherry Chipotle Bbq Chicken Wings

Servings: 2
Cooking Time: 12 Minutes

Ingredients:

- 1 teaspoon smoked paprika
- ½ teaspoon dry mustard powder
- 1 teaspoon dried oregano
- 1 teaspoon dried thyme
- ½ teaspoon chili powder
- 1 teaspoon salt
- 2 pounds chicken wings
- vegetable oil or spray
- salt and freshly ground black pepper
- 1 to 2 tablespoons chopped chipotle peppers in adobo sauce
- ⅓ cup cherry preserves ¼ cup tomato ketchup

Directions:

1. Combine the first six ingredients in a large bowl. Prepare the chicken wings by cutting off the wing tips and discarding (or freezing for chicken stock). Divide the drumettes from the win-gettes by cutting through the joint. Place the chicken wing pieces in the bowl with the spice mix. Toss or shake well to coat.

2. Preheat the toaster oven to 400°F.

3. Spray the wings lightly with the vegetable oil and air-fry the wings in two batches for 10 minutes per batch. When both batches are done, toss all the wings back into the air fryer oven for

another 2 minutes to heat through and finish cooking.

4. While the wings are air-frying, combine the chopped chipotle peppers, cherry preserves and ketchup in a bowl.

5. Remove the wings from the air fryer oven, toss them in the cherry chipotle BBQ sauce and serve with napkins!

Buffalo Cauliflower

Servings: 4
Cooking Time: 30 Minutes

Ingredients:

- 1 cup gluten free panko breadcrumbs
- 1 teaspoon ground paprika
- ½ teaspoon garlic powder
- ¼ teaspoon onion powder
- ½ teaspoon cayenne pepper
- 1 teaspoon kosher salt
- ½ teaspoon freshly ground black pepper
- 1 head cauliflower, cut into florets
- 2 tablespoons cornstarch
- 3 eggs, beaten
- Cooking spray
- ¾ cup buffalo wing sauce, warm
- Ranch or bleu cheese dressing, for serving

Directions:

1. Combine panko breadcrumbs, paprika, garlic powder, onion powder, cayenne pepper, kosher salt, and black pepper in a large bowl. Set aside.

2. Toss together cauliflower and cornstarch until the cauliflower is lightly coated.

3. Shake any excess cornstarch off the cauliflower, then dip into beaten eggs, then into seasoned breadcrumbs.

4. Spray the breaded cauliflower with cooking spray, place into the fry basket, and set aside. You may need to work in batches.

5. Preheat the toaster oven to 380°F.

6. Insert the fry basket with the cauliflower at top position in the preheated oven.

7. Select the Air Fry and Shake functions, adjust time to 30 minutes, and press Start/Pause.

8. Flip the cauliflower halfway through cooking. The Shake Reminder will let you know when.

9. Remove when done and place into a large bowl.

10. Toss the cauliflower in the buffalo wing sauce until they are well coated.

11. Serve with a side of ranch or blue cheese dressing.

Warm And Salty Edamame

Servings: 4
Cooking Time: 10 Minutes

Ingredients:

- 1 pound Unshelled edamame
- Vegetable oil spray
- ¾ teaspoon Coarse sea salt or kosher salt

Directions:

1. Preheat the toaster oven to 400°F.

2. Place the edamame in a large bowl and lightly coat them with vegetable oil spray. Toss well, spray again, and toss until they are evenly coated.

3. When the machine is at temperature, pour the edamame into the air fryer oven and air-fry, tossing the pan quite often to rearrange the edamame, for 7 minutes, or until warm and aromatic. (Air-fry for 10 minutes if the edamame were frozen and not thawed.)

4. Pour the edamame into a bowl and sprinkle the salt on top. Toss well, then set aside for a couple of minutes before serving with an empty bowl on the side for the pods.

FISH AND SEAFOOD

Fish Tacos With Jalapeño-lime Sauce

Servings: 4
Cooking Time: 7 Minutes

Ingredients:

- Fish Tacos
- 1 pound fish fillets
- ¼ teaspoon cumin
- ¼ teaspoon coriander
- ⅛ teaspoon ground red pepper
- 1 tablespoon lime zest
- ¼ teaspoon smoked paprika
- 1 teaspoon oil
- cooking spray
- 6–8 corn or flour tortillas (6-inch size)
- Jalapeño-Lime Sauce
- ½ cup sour cream
- 1 tablespoon lime juice
- ¼ teaspoon grated lime zest
- ½ teaspoon minced jalapeño (flesh only)
- ¼ teaspoon cumin
- Napa Cabbage Garnish
- 1 cup shredded Napa cabbage
- ¼ cup slivered red or green bell pepper
- ¼ cup slivered onion

Directions:

1. Slice the fish fillets into strips approximately ½-inch thick.
2. Put the strips into a sealable plastic bag along with the cumin, coriander, red pepper, lime zest, smoked paprika, and oil. Massage seasonings into the fish until evenly distributed.
3. Spray air fryer oven with nonstick cooking spray and place seasoned fish inside.

4. Air-fry at 390°F for approximately 5 minutes. Distribute fish. Cook an additional 2 minutes, until fish flakes easily.
5. While the fish is cooking, prepare the Jalapeño-Lime Sauce by mixing the sour cream, lime juice, lime zest, jalapeño, and cumin together to make a smooth sauce. Set aside.
6. Mix the cabbage, bell pepper, and onion together and set aside.
7. To warm refrigerated tortillas, wrap in damp paper towels and microwave for 30 to 60 seconds.
8. To serve, spoon some of fish into a warm tortilla. Add one or two tablespoons Napa Cabbage Garnish and drizzle with Jalapeño-Lime Sauce.

Crispy Sweet-and-sour Cod Fillets

Servings: 3
Cooking Time: 12 Minutes

Ingredients:

- 1½ cups Plain panko bread crumbs (gluten-free, if a concern)
- 2 tablespoons Regular or low-fat mayonnaise (not fat-free; gluten-free, if a concern)
- ¼ cup Sweet pickle relish
- 3 4- to 5-ounce skinless cod fillets

Directions:

1. Preheat the toaster oven to 400°F.
2. Pour the bread crumbs into a shallow soup plate or a small pie plate. Mix the mayonnaise and relish in a small bowl until well combined. Smear this mixture all over the cod fillets. Set them in the crumbs and turn until evenly coated on all sides, even on the ends.

3. Set the coated cod fillets in the air fryer oven with as much air space between them as possible. They should not touch. Air-fry undisturbed for 12 minutes, or until browned and crisp.

4. Use a nonstick-safe spatula to transfer the cod pieces to a wire rack. Cool for only a minute or two before serving hot.

Snapper With Capers And Olives

Servings: 2

Cooking Time: 10 Minutes

Ingredients:

- 2 tablespoons capers
- ¼ cup pitted and sliced black olives
- 2 tablespoons olive oil
- ½ teaspoon dried oregano
- Salt and freshly ground black pepper to taste
- 2 6-ounce red snapper fillets
- 1 tomato, cut into wedges

Directions:

1. Combine the capers, olives, olive oil, and seasonings in a bowl.

2. Place the fillets in an oiled or nonstick 8½ × 8½ × 2-inch square baking (cake) pan and spoon the caper mixture over them.

3. BROIL for 10 minutes, or until the fish flakes easily with a fork. Serve with the tomato wedges.

Flounder Fillets

Servings: 4

Cooking Time: 8 Minutes

Ingredients:

- 1 egg white
- 1 tablespoon water
- 1 cup panko breadcrumbs
- 2 tablespoons extra-light virgin olive oil
- 4 4-ounce flounder fillets
- salt and pepper

- oil for misting or cooking spray

Directions:

1. Preheat the toaster oven to 390°F.

2. Beat together egg white and water in shallow dish.

3. In another shallow dish, mix panko crumbs and oil until well combined and crumbly (best done by hand).

4. Season flounder fillets with salt and pepper to taste. Dip each fillet into egg mixture and then roll in panko crumbs, pressing in crumbs so that fish is nicely coated.

5. Spray air fryer oven with nonstick cooking spray and add fillets. Air-fry at 390°F for 3 minutes.

6. Spray fish fillets but do not turn. Cook 5 minutes longer or until golden brown and crispy. Using a spatula, carefully remove fish from air fryer oven and serve.

Better Fish Sticks

Servings: 3

Cooking Time: 8 Minutes

Ingredients:

- ¾ cup Seasoned Italian-style dried bread crumbs (gluten-free, if a concern)
- 3 tablespoons (about ½ ounce) Finely grated Parmesan cheese
- 10 ounces Skinless cod fillets, cut lengthwise into 1-inch-wide pieces
- 3 tablespoons Regular or low-fat mayonnaise (not fat-free; gluten-free, if a concern)
- Vegetable oil spray

Directions:

1. Preheat the toaster oven to 400°F.

2. Mix the bread crumbs and grated Parmesan in a shallow soup bowl or a small pie plate.

3. Smear the fish fillet sticks completely with the mayonnaise, then dip them one by one in the bread-crumb mixture, turning and pressing gently to make an even and thorough coating. Coat each stick on all sides with vegetable oil spray.

4. Set the fish sticks in the air fryer oven with at least ¼ inch between them. Air-fry undisturbed for 8 minutes, or until golden brown and crisp.

5. Use a nonstick-safe spatula to gently transfer them from the air fryer oven to a wire rack. Cool for only a minute or two before serving.

Quick Shrimp Scampi

Servings: 2
Cooking Time: 5 Minutes

Ingredients:

- 16 to 20 raw large shrimp, peeled, deveined and tails removed
- ½ cup white wine
- freshly ground black pepper
- ¼ cup + 1 tablespoon butter, divided
- 1 clove garlic, sliced
- 1 teaspoon olive oil
- salt, to taste
- juice of ½ lemon, to taste
- ¼ cup chopped fresh parsley

Directions:

1. Start by marinating the shrimp in the white wine and freshly ground black pepper for at least 30 minutes, or as long as 2 hours in the refrigerator.

2. Preheat the toaster oven to 400°F.

3. Melt ¼ cup of butter in a small saucepan on the stovetop. Add the garlic and let the butter simmer, but be sure to not let it burn.

4. Pour the shrimp and marinade into the air fryer oven, letting the marinade drain through to the bottom drawer. Drizzle the olive oil on the shrimp and season well with salt. Air-fry at 400°F for 3 minutes. Turn the shrimp over and pour the garlic butter over the shrimp. Air-fry for another 2 minutes.

5. Remove the shrimp from the air fryer oven and transfer them to a bowl. Squeeze lemon juice over all the shrimp and toss with the chopped parsley and remaining tablespoon of butter. Season to taste with salt and serve immediately.

Garlic-lemon Shrimp Skewers

Servings: 2
Cooking Time: 8 Minutes

Ingredients:

- Juice and zest of 1 lemon
- 1 tablespoon olive oil
- ½ teaspoon garlic puree
- ¼ teaspoon smoked paprika
- 12 large shrimp, peeled and deveined
- Oil spray (hand-pumped)
- Sea salt, for seasoning
- Freshly ground black pepper, for seasoning
- 1 tablespoon chopped fresh parsley

Directions:

1. Preheat the toaster oven to 350°F on AIR FRY for 5 minutes.

2. In a medium bowl, stir the lemon juice, lemon zest, olive oil, garlic, and paprika.

3. Add the shrimp and toss to combine. Cover, refrigerate, and let marinate for 30 minutes.

4. Soak 4 wooden skewers in water while the shrimp marinate.

5. Place the air-fryer basket in the baking tray and spray it generously with the oil.

6. Thread 3 shrimp on each skewer and place them in the basket. Discard any remaining marinade.

7. In position 2, air fry for 8 minutes, turning halfway through, until just cooked.

8. Season with the salt and pepper and serve topped with the parsley.

Blackened Red Snapper

Servings: 4
Cooking Time: 8 Minutes

Ingredients:
- 1½ teaspoons black pepper
- ¼ teaspoon thyme
- ¼ teaspoon garlic powder
- ⅛ teaspoon cayenne pepper
- 1 teaspoon olive oil
- 4 4-ounce red snapper fillet portions, skin on
- 4 thin slices lemon
- cooking spray

Directions:
1. Mix the spices and oil together to make a paste. Rub into both sides of the fish.

2. Spray air fryer oven with nonstick cooking spray and lay snapper steaks in air fryer oven, skin-side down.

3. Place a lemon slice on each piece of fish.

4. Air-fry at 390°F for 8 minutes. The fish will not flake when done, but it should be white through the center.

Crab-stuffed Peppers

Servings: 4
Cooking Time: 45 Minutes

Ingredients:
- Filling:
- 1½ cups fresh crabmeat, chopped, or 2 6-ounce cans lump crabmeat, drained
- 4 plum tomatoes, chopped
- 2 4-ounce cans sliced mushrooms, drained well

- 4 tablespoons pitted and sliced black olives
- 2 tablespoons olive oil
- 2 garlic cloves, minced
- ½ teaspoon ground cumin
- Salt and freshly ground black pepper to taste
- 4 large bell peppers, tops cut off, seeds and membrane removed
- ½ cup shredded low-fat mozzarella cheese

Directions:
1. Preheat the toaster oven to 375° F.

2. Combine the filling ingredients in a bowl and adjust the seasonings. Spoon the mixture to generously fill each pepper. Place the peppers upright in an 8½ × 8½ × 2-inch oiled or nonstick square (cake) pan.

3. BAKE for 40 minutes, or until the peppers are tender. Remove from the oven and sprinkle the cheese in equal portions on top of the peppers.

4. BROIL 5 minutes, or until the cheese is melted.

Crunchy And Buttery Cod With Ritz® Cracker Crust

Servings: 2
Cooking Time: 10 Minutes

Ingredients:
- 4 tablespoons butter, melted
- 8 to 10 RITZ® crackers, crushed into crumbs
- 2 (6-ounce) cod fillets
- salt and freshly ground black pepper
- 1 lemon

Directions:
1. Preheat the toaster oven to 380°F.

2. Melt the butter in a small saucepan on the stovetop or in a microwavable dish in the microwave, and then transfer the butter to a shallow dish. Place the crushed RITZ® crackers into a second shallow dish.

3. Season the fish fillets with salt and freshly ground black pepper. Dip them into the butter and then coat both sides with the RITZ® crackers.
4. Place the fish into the air fryer oven and air-fry at 380°F for 10 minutes, flipping the fish over halfway through the cooking time.
5. Serve with a wedge of lemon to squeeze over the top.

Fish Sticks For Kids

Servings: 8
Cooking Time: 6 Minutes

Ingredients:
- 8 ounces fish fillets (pollock or cod)
- salt (optional)
- ½ cup plain breadcrumbs
- oil for misting or cooking spray

Directions:
1. Cut fish fillets into "fingers" about ½ x 3 inches. Sprinkle with salt to taste, if desired.
2. Roll fish in breadcrumbs. Spray all sides with oil or cooking spray.
3. Place in air fryer oven in single layer and air-fry at 390°F for 6 minutes, until golden brown and crispy.

Baked Clam Appetizers

Servings: 12
Cooking Time: 10 Minutes

Ingredients:
- 1 6-ounce can minced clams, well drained
- 1 cup multigrain bread crumbs
- 1 tablespoon minced onion
- 1 teaspoon garlic powder
- 1 teaspoon Worcestershire sauce
- 1 tablespoon chopped fresh parsley
- 2 tablespoons olive oil
- Salt and freshly ground black pepper
- Lemon wedges

Directions:
1. Preheat the toaster oven to 450° F.
2. Combine all the ingredients in a medium bowl and fill 12 scrubbed clamshells or small baking dishes with equal portions of the mixture. Place in an 8½ × 8½ × 2-inch oiled or nonstick square (cake) pan.
3. BAKE for 10 minutes, or until lightly browned.

Maple Balsamic Glazed Salmon

Servings: 4
Cooking Time: 10 Minutes

Ingredients:
- 4 (6-ounce) fillets of salmon
- salt and freshly ground black pepper
- vegetable oil
- ¼ cup pure maple syrup
- 3 tablespoons balsamic vinegar
- 1 teaspoon Dijon mustard

Directions:
1. Preheat the toaster oven to 400°F.
2. Season the salmon well with salt and freshly ground black pepper. Spray or brush the bottom of the air fryer oven with vegetable oil and place the salmon fillets inside. Air-fry the salmon for 5 minutes.
3. While the salmon is air-frying, combine the maple syrup, balsamic vinegar and Dijon mustard in a small saucepan over medium heat and stir to blend well. Let the mixture simmer while the fish is cooking. It should start to thicken slightly, but keep your eye on it so it doesn't burn.
4. Brush the glaze on the salmon fillets and air-fry for an additional 5 minutes. The salmon should feel firm to the touch when finished and the glaze should be nicely browned on top. Brush a little more glaze on top before removing and serving with rice and vegetables, or a nice green salad.

Fish With Sun-dried Tomato Pesto

Servings: 4
Cooking Time: 31 Minutes

Ingredients:
- Tomato sauce:
- ¼ cup chopped sun-dried tomatoes
- 2 tablespoons chopped fresh basil
- ⅔ cup dry white wine
- 2 tablespoons grated Parmesan cheese
- 2 tablespoons olive oil
- 1 tablespoon pine nuts
- 2 garlic cloves
- Salt and freshly ground black pepper to taste
- 4 6-ounce fish fillets (trout, catfish, flounder, or tilapia)
- 1 tablespoon reduced-fat mayonnaise
- 2 tablespoons chopped fresh cilantro Olive oil

Directions:
1. Preheat the toaster oven to 400° F.
2. Process the tomato sauce ingredients in a blender or food processor until smooth.
3. Layer the fish fillets in an oiled or nonstick 8½ × 8½ × 2-inch square baking (cake) pan. Spoon the sauce over the fish, spreading evenly.
4. BAKE, uncovered, for 25 minutes, or until the fish flakes easily with a fork. Remove from the oven, spread the mayonnaise on top of the fish, and garnish with the cilantro.
5. BROIL for 6 minutes, or until lightly browned.

Oven-poached Salmon

Servings: 2
Cooking Time: 20 Minutes

Ingredients:
- Poaching liquid:
- 1 cup dry white wine
- 2 bay leaves
- 1 tablespoon mustard seed
- Salt and freshly ground black pepper to taste
- 2 6-ounce salmon steaks
- 2 tablespoons fresh watercress, rinsed, drained, and chopped (for serving hot)
- 1 lemon, cut into small wedges (for serving hot)
- Cucumber Sauce (recipe follows)

Directions:
1. Preheat the toaster oven to 350° F.
2. Combine the poaching liquid ingredients with 1 cup water in a small bowl and set aside.
3. Place the salmon steaks in an oiled or nonstick 8½ × 8½ × 2-inch square baking (cake) pan and pour enough poaching liquid over the steaks to barely cover them. Adjust the seasonings to taste.
4. BAKE, uncovered, for 20 minutes, or until the fish feels springy to the touch. Remove the bay leaves and serve the fish hot with watercress and lemon or cold with Cucumber Sauce.

Butternut Squash–wrapped Halibut Fillets

Servings: 3
Cooking Time: 11 Minutes

Ingredients:
- 15 Long spiralized peeled and seeded butternut squash strands
- 3 5- to 6-ounce skinless halibut fillets
- 3 tablespoons Butter, melted
- ¾ teaspoon Mild paprika
- ¾ teaspoon Table salt
- ¾ teaspoon Ground black pepper

Directions:
1. Preheat the toaster oven to 375°F .

2. Hold 5 long butternut squash strands together and wrap them around a fillet. Set it aside and wrap any remaining fillet(s).

3. Mix the melted butter, paprika, salt, and pepper in a small bowl. Brush this mixture over the squash-wrapped fillets on all sides.

4. When the machine is at temperature, set the fillets in the air fryer oven with as much air space between them as possible. Air-fry undisturbed for 10 minutes, or until the squash strands have browned but not burned. If the machine is at 360°F, you may need to add 1 minute to the cooking time. In any event, watch the fish carefully after the 8-minute mark.

5. Use a nonstick-safe spatula to gently transfer the fillets to a serving platter or plates. Cool for only a minute or so before serving.

Fried Scallops

Servings: 3
Cooking Time: 6 Minutes

Ingredients:
- ½ cup All-purpose flour or tapioca flour
- 1 Large egg(s), well beaten
- 2 cups Corn flake crumbs (gluten-free, if a concern)
- Up to 2 teaspoons Cayenne
- 1 teaspoon Celery seeds
- 1 teaspoon Table salt
- 1 pound Sea scallops
- Vegetable oil spray

Directions:
1. Preheat the toaster oven to 400°F.

2. Set up and fill three shallow soup plates or small pie plates on your counter: one for the flour; one for the beaten egg(s); and one for the corn flake crumbs, stirred with the cayenne, celery seeds, and salt until well combined.

3. One by one, dip a scallop in the flour, turning it every way to coat it thoroughly. Gently shake off any excess flour, then dip the scallop in the egg(s), turning it again to coat all sides. Let any excess egg slip back into the rest, then set the scallop in the corn flake mixture. Turn it several times, pressing gently to get an even coating on the scallop all around. Generously coat the scallop with vegetable oil spray, then set it aside on a cutting board. Coat the remaining scallops in the same way.

4. Set the scallops in the air fryer oven with as much air space between them as possible. They should not touch. Air-fry undisturbed for 6 minutes, or until lightly browned and firm.

5. Use kitchen tongs to gently transfer the scallops to a wire rack. Cool for only a minute or two before serving.

Horseradish-crusted Salmon Fillets

Servings: 3
Cooking Time: 8 Minutes

Ingredients:
- ½ cup Fresh bread crumbs
- 4 tablespoons (¼ cup/½ stick) Butter, melted and cooled
- ¼ cup Jarred prepared white horseradish
- Vegetable oil spray
- 4 6-ounce skin-on salmon fillets

Directions:
1. Preheat the toaster oven to 400°F.

2. Mix the bread crumbs, butter, and horseradish in a bowl until well combined.

3. Take the pan out of the machine. Generously spray the skin side of each fillet. Pick them up one by one with a nonstick-safe spatula and set them in the pan skin side down with as much air

space between them as possible. Divide the bread-crumb mixture between the fillets, coating the top of each fillet with an even layer. Generously coat the bread-crumb mixture with vegetable oil spray.

4. Return the pan to the machine and air-fry undisturbed for 8 minutes, or until the topping has lightly browned and the fish is firm but not hard.

5. Use a nonstick-safe spatula to transfer the salmon fillets to serving plates. Cool for 5 minutes before serving. Because of the butter in the topping, it will stay very hot for quite a while. Take care, especially if you're serving these fillets to children.

Stuffed Shrimp

Servings: 4
Cooking Time: 12 Minutes

Ingredients:

- 16 tail-on shrimp, peeled and deveined (last tail section intact)
- ¾ cup crushed panko breadcrumbs
- oil for misting or cooking spray
- Stuffing
- 2 6-ounce cans lump crabmeat
- 2 tablespoons chopped shallots
- 2 tablespoons chopped green onions
- 2 tablespoons chopped celery
- 2 tablespoons chopped green bell pepper
- ½ cup crushed saltine crackers
- 1 teaspoon Old Bay Seasoning
- 1 teaspoon garlic powder
- ¼ teaspoon ground thyme
- 2 teaspoons dried parsley flakes
- 2 teaspoons fresh lemon juice
- 2 teaspoons Worcestershire sauce
- 1 egg, beaten

Directions:

1. Rinse shrimp. Remove tail section (shell) from 4 shrimp, discard, and chop the meat finely.

2. To prepare the remaining 12 shrimp, cut a deep slit down the back side so that the meat lies open flat. Do not cut all the way through.

3. Preheat the toaster oven to 360°F.

4. Place chopped shrimp in a large bowl with all of the stuffing ingredients and stir to combine.

5. Divide stuffing into 12 portions, about 2 tablespoons each.

6. Place one stuffing portion onto the back of each shrimp and form into a ball or oblong shape. Press firmly so that stuffing sticks together and adheres to shrimp.

7. Gently roll each stuffed shrimp in panko crumbs and mist with oil or cooking spray.

8. Place 6 shrimp in air fryer oven and air-fry at 360°F for 10 minutes. Mist with oil or spray and cook 2 minutes longer or until stuffing cooks through inside and is crispy outside.

9. Repeat step 8 to cook remaining shrimp.

Shrimp With Jalapeño Dip

Servings: 4
Cooking Time: 10 Minutes

Ingredients:

- Seasonings:
- 1 teaspoon ground cumin
- 1 tablespoon minced garlic
- 1 teaspoon paprika
- 1 teaspoon chili powder
- Pinch of cayenne
- Salt to taste
- 1½ pounds large shrimp, peeled and deveined

Directions:

1. Combine the seasonings in a plastic bag, add the shrimp, and shake well to coat. Transfer the

shrimp to an oiled or nonstick 8½ × 8½ × 2-inch square baking (cake) pan.

2. BROIL for 5 minutes. Remove the pan from the oven and turn the shrimp with tongs. Broil 5 minutes again, or until the shrimp are cooked (they should be firm but not rubbery.) Serve with Jalapeño Dip.

Broiled Scallops

Servings: 6
Cooking Time: 3 Minutes

Ingredients:
- Broiling sauce:
- 2 tablespoons chopped fresh parsley
- 3 shallots, finely chopped
- ¾ cup white wine
- 3 tablespoons margarine, at room
- Temperature
- ½ teaspoon dried thyme
- 3 tablespoons sesame seeds
- Salt and freshly ground black pepper
- 1½ pounds (3 cups) bay scallops, rinsed and drained

Directions:
1. Whisk together the ingredients for the broiling sauce in a small bowl and transfer to a 1-quart 8½ × 8½ × 4-inch ovenproof baking dish. Adjust the seasoning, add the scallops, and spoon the mixture over them.

2. BROIL for 3 minutes, or until all the scallops are opaque instead of translucent. Serve with the sauce.

Best-dressed Trout

Servings: 2
Cooking Time: 25 Minutes

Ingredients:
- 2 dressed trout

- 1 egg, beaten
- 2 tablespoons finely ground almonds
- 2 tablespoons unbleached flour
- 1 teaspoon paprika or smoked paprika
- Pinch of salt (optional)
- 4 lemon slices, approximately ¼ inch thick
- 1 teaspoon lemon juice

Directions:
1. Preheat the toaster oven to 400° F.

2. Brush the trout (both sides) with the beaten egg. Blend the almonds, flour, paprika, and salt in a bowl and sprinkle both sides of the trout. Insert 2 lemon slices in each trout cavity and place the trout in an oiled or nonstick 8½ × 8½ × 2-inch square baking (cake) pan.

3. BAKE for 20 minutes, or until the meat is white and firm. Remove from the oven and turn the trout carefully with a spatula.

4. BROIL for 5 minutes, or until the trout is lightly browned.

Horseradish Crusted Salmon

Servings: 2
Cooking Time: 14 Minutes

Ingredients:
- 2 (5-ounce) salmon fillets
- salt and freshly ground black pepper
- 2 teaspoons Dijon mustard
- ½ cup panko breadcrumbs
- 2 tablespoons prepared horseradish
- ½ teaspoon finely chopped lemon zest
- 1 tablespoon olive oil
- 1 tablespoon chopped fresh parsley

Directions:
1. Preheat the toaster oven to 360°F.

2. Season the salmon with salt and freshly ground black pepper. Then spread the Dijon mustard on the salmon, coating the entire surface.

3. Combine the breadcrumbs, horseradish, lemon zest and olive oil in a small bowl. Spread the mixture over the top of the salmon and press down lightly with your hands, adhering it to the salmon using the mustard as "glue".

4. Transfer the salmon to the air fryer oven and air-fry at 360°F for 14 minutes (depending on how thick your fillet is) or until the fish feels firm to the touch. Sprinkle with the parsley.

Marinated Catfish

Servings: 4

Cooking Time: 10 Minutes

Ingredients:

- Marinade:
- 1 tablespoon olive oil
- 1 tablespoon lemon juice
- ¼ dry white wine
- 1 tablespoon garlic powder
- 1 tablespoon soy sauce
- 4 6-ounce catfish fillets

Directions:

1. Combine the marinade ingredients in an 8½ × 8½ × 4-inch ovenproof baking dish. Add the fillets and let stand for 10 minutes, spooning the marinade over the fillets every 2 minutes.

2. BROIL the fillets for 15 minutes, or until the fish flakes easily with a fork.

Sweet Chili Shrimp

Servings: 4

Cooking Time: 6 Minutes

Ingredients:

- 1 pound jumbo shrimp, peeled and deveined
- ¼ cup sweet chili sauce
- 1 lime, zested and juiced
- 1 tablespoon soy sauce
- 1 tablespoon honey
- 1 tablespoon olive oil
- 1 large garlic clove, minced
- ½ teaspoon salt
- ¼ teaspoon pepper
- 1 green onion, thinly sliced, for garnish

Directions:

1. Place the shrimp in a large bowl. Whisk all the remaining ingredients except the green onion in a separate bowl.

2. Pour sauce over the shrimp and toss to coat.

3. Preheat the toaster Oven to 430°F.

4. Line the food tray with foil, place shrimp on the tray, then insert at top position in the preheated oven.

5. Select the Air Fry function, adjust time to 6 minutes, and press Start/Pause.

6. Remove shrimp and garnish with sliced green onions.

Almond-crusted Fish

Servings: 4

Cooking Time: 10 Minutes

Ingredients:

- 4 4-ounce fish fillets
- ¾ cup breadcrumbs
- ¼ cup sliced almonds, crushed
- 2 tablespoons lemon juice
- ⅛ teaspoon cayenne
- salt and pepper
- ¾ cup flour
- 1 egg, beaten with 1 tablespoon water
- oil for misting or cooking spray

Directions:

1. Split fish fillets lengthwise down the center to create 8 pieces.

2. Mix breadcrumbs and almonds together and set aside.

3. Mix the lemon juice and cayenne together. Brush on all sides of fish.

4. Season fish to taste with salt and pepper.

5. Place the flour on a sheet of wax paper.

6. Roll fillets in flour, dip in egg wash, and roll in the crumb mixture.

7. Mist both sides of fish with oil or cooking spray.

8. Spray air fryer oven and lay fillets inside.

9. Air-fry at 390°F for 5 minutes, turn fish over, and air-fry for an additional 5 minutes or until fish is done and flakes easily.

BEEF PORK AND LAMB

Skirt Steak Fajitas

Servings: 4
Cooking Time: 30 Minutes

Ingredients:

- 2 tablespoons olive oil
- ¼ cup lime juice
- 1 clove garlic, minced
- ½ teaspoon ground cumin
- ½ teaspoon hot sauce
- ½ teaspoon salt
- 2 tablespoons chopped fresh cilantro
- 1 pound skirt steak
- 1 onion, sliced
- 1 teaspoon chili powder
- 1 red pepper, sliced
- 1 green pepper, sliced
- salt and freshly ground black pepper
- 8 flour tortillas
- shredded lettuce, crumbled Queso Fresco (or grated Cheddar cheese), sliced black olives, diced tomatoes, sour cream and guacamole for serving

Directions:

1. Combine the olive oil, lime juice, garlic, cumin, hot sauce, salt and cilantro in a shallow dish. Add the skirt steak and turn it over several times to coat all sides. Pierce the steak with a needle-style meat tenderizer or paring knife. Marinate the steak in the refrigerator for at least 3 hours, or overnight. When you are ready to cook, remove the steak from the refrigerator and let it sit at room temperature for 30 minutes.
2. Preheat the toaster oven to 400°F.
3. Toss the onion slices with the chili powder and a little olive oil and transfer them to the air fryer oven. Air-fry at 400°F for 5 minutes. Add the red and green peppers to the air fryer oven with the onions, season with salt and pepper and air-fry for 8 more minutes, until the onions and peppers are soft. Transfer the vegetables to a dish and cover with aluminum foil to keep warm.
4. Place the skirt steak in the air fryer oven and pour the marinade over the top. Air-fry at 400°F for 12 minutes. Flip the steak over and air-fry at 400°F for an additional 5 minutes. (The time needed for your steak will depend on the thickness of the skirt steak. 17 minutes should bring your steak to roughly medium.) Transfer the cooked steak to a cutting board and let the steak rest for a few minutes. If the peppers and onions need to be heated, return them to the air fryer oven for just 1 to 2 minutes.
5. Thinly slice the steak at an angle, cutting against the grain of the steak. Serve the steak with the onions and peppers, the warm tortillas and the fajita toppings on the side so that everyone can make their own fajita.

Italian Meatballs

Servings: 4
Cooking Time: 12 Minutes

Ingredients:

- 12 ounces lean ground beef
- 4 ounces Italian sausage, casing removed
- ½ cup breadcrumbs
- 1 cup grated Parmesan cheese
- 1 egg
- 2 tablespoons milk
- 2 teaspoons Italian seasoning
- ½ teaspoon onion powder
- ½ teaspoon garlic powder
- Pinch of red pepper flakes

Directions:

1. In a large bowl, place all the ingredients and mix well. Roll out 24 meatballs.

2. Preheat the toaster oven to 360°F.

3. Place the meatballs in the air fryer oven and air-fry for 12 minutes, tossing every 4 minutes. Using a food thermometer, check to ensure the internal temperature of the meatballs is 165°F.

Calzones South Of The Border

Servings: 8

Cooking Time: 8 Minutes

Ingredients:

- Filling
- ¼ pound ground pork sausage
- ½ teaspoon chile powder
- ¼ teaspoon ground cumin
- ⅛ teaspoon garlic powder
- ⅛ teaspoon onion powder
- ⅛ teaspoon oregano
- ½ cup ricotta cheese
- 1 ounce sharp Cheddar cheese, shredded
- 2 ounces Pepper Jack cheese, shredded
- 1 4-ounce can chopped green chiles, drained
- oil for misting or cooking spray
- salsa, sour cream, or guacamole
- Crust
- 2 cups white wheat flour, plus more for kneading and rolling
- 1 package (¼ ounce) RapidRise yeast
- 1 teaspoon salt
- ½ teaspoon chile powder
- ½ teaspoon ground cumin
- 1 cup warm water (115°F to 125°F)
- 2 teaspoons olive oil

Directions:

1. Crumble sausage into air fryer oven baking pan and stir in the filling seasonings: chile powder, cumin, garlic powder, onion powder, and oregano. Air-fry at 390°F for 2 minutes. Stir, breaking apart, and air-fry for 3 to 4 minutes, until well done. Remove and set aside on paper towels to drain.

2. To make dough, combine flour, yeast, salt, chile powder, and cumin. Stir in warm water and oil until soft dough forms. Turn out onto lightly floured board and knead for 3 or 4 minutes. Let dough rest for 10 minutes.

3. Place the three cheeses in a medium bowl. Add cooked sausage and chiles and stir until well mixed.

4. Cut dough into 8 pieces.

5. Working with 4 pieces of the dough, press each into a circle about 5 inches in diameter. Top each dough circle with 2 heaping tablespoons of filling. Fold over into a half-moon shape and press edges together. Seal edges firmly to prevent leakage. Spray both sides with oil or cooking spray.

6. Place 4 calzones in air fryer oven and air-fry at 360°F for 5 minutes. Mist with oil or spray and air-fry for 3 minutes, until crust is done and nicely browned.

7. While the first batch is cooking, press out the remaining dough, fill, and shape into calzones.

8. Spray both sides with oil or cooking spray and air-fry for 5 minutes. If needed, mist with oil and continue cooking for 3 minutes longer. This second batch will cook a little faster than the first because your air fryer oven is already hot.

9. Serve plain or with salsa, sour cream, or guacamole.

Crunchy Fried Pork Loin Chops

Servings: 3

Cooking Time: 12 Minutes

Ingredients:

- 1 cup All-purpose flour or tapioca flour
- 1 Large egg(s), well beaten
- 1½ cups Seasoned Italian-style dried bread crumbs (gluten-free, if a concern)
- 3 4- to 5-ounce boneless center-cut pork loin chops
- Vegetable oil spray

Directions:

1. Preheat the toaster oven to 350°F .

2. Set up and fill three shallow soup plates or small pie plates on your counter: one for the flour, one for the beaten egg(s), and one for the bread crumbs.

3. Dredge a pork chop in the flour, coating both sides as well as around the edge. Gently shake off any excess, then dip the chop in the egg(s), again coating both sides and the edge. Let any excess egg slip back into the rest, then set the chop in the bread crumbs, turning it and pressing gently to coat well on both sides and the edge. Coat the pork chop all over with vegetable oil spray and set aside so you can dredge, coat, and spray the additional chop(s).

4. Set the chops in the air fryer oven with as much air space between them as possible. Air-fry undisturbed for 12 minutes, or until brown and crunchy and an instant-read meat thermometer inserted into the center of a chop registers 145°F.

5. Use kitchen tongs to transfer the chops to a wire rack. Cool for 5 minutes before serving.

Pretzel-coated Pork Tenderloin

Servings: 4

Cooking Time: 10 Minutes

Ingredients:

- 1 Large egg white(s)
- 2 teaspoons Dijon mustard (gluten-free, if a concern)
- 1½ cups (about 6 ounces) Crushed pretzel crumbs
- 1 pound (4 sections) Pork tenderloin, cut into ¼-pound (4-ounce) sections
- Vegetable oil spray

Directions:

1. Preheat the toaster oven to 350°F .

2. Set up and fill two shallow soup plates or small pie plates on your counter: one for the egg white(s), whisked with the mustard until foamy; and one for the pretzel crumbs.

3. Dip a section of pork tenderloin in the egg white mixture and turn it to coat well, even on the ends. Let any excess egg white mixture slip back into the rest, then set the pork in the pretzel crumbs. Roll it several times, pressing gently, until the pork is evenly coated, even on the ends. Generously coat the pork section with vegetable oil spray, set it aside, and continue coating and spraying the remaining sections.

4. Set the pork sections in the air fryer oven with at least ¼ inch between them. Air-fry undisturbed for 10 minutes, or until an instant-read meat thermometer inserted into the center of one section registers 145°F.

5. Use kitchen tongs to transfer the pieces to a wire rack. Cool for 3 to 5 minutes before serving.

Seasoned Boneless Pork Sirloin Chops

Servings: 2

Cooking Time: 16 Minutes

Ingredients:

- Seasoning mixture:

- ½ teaspoon ground cumin
- ¼ teaspoon turmeric
- Pinch of ground cardamom
- Pinch of grated nutmeg
- 1 teaspoon vegetable oil
- 1 teaspoon Pickapeppa sauce
- 2½- to ¾-pound boneless lean pork sirloin chops

Directions:

1. Combine the seasoning mixture ingredients in a small bowl and brush on both sides of the chops. Place the chops on the broiling rack with a pan underneath.

2. BROIL 8 minutes, remove the chops, turn, and brush with the mixture. Broil again for 8 minutes, or until the chops are done to your preference.

Italian Sausage & Peppers

Servings: 6
Cooking Time: 25 Minutes

Ingredients:

- 1 6-ounce can tomato paste
- ⅔ cup water
- 1 8-ounce can tomato sauce
- 1 teaspoon dried parsley flakes
- ½ teaspoon garlic powder
- ⅛ teaspoon oregano
- ½ pound mild Italian bulk sausage
- 1 tablespoon extra virgin olive oil
- ½ large onion, cut in 1-inch chunks
- 4 ounces fresh mushrooms, sliced
- 1 large green bell pepper, cut in 1-inch chunks
- 8 ounces spaghetti, cooked
- Parmesan cheese for serving

Directions:

1. In a large saucepan or skillet, stir together the tomato paste, water, tomato sauce, parsley, garlic, and oregano. Heat on stovetop over very low heat while preparing meat and vegetables.

2. Break sausage into small chunks, about ½-inch pieces. Place in air fryer oven baking pan.

3. Air-fry at 390°F for 5 minutes. Stir. Cook 7 minutes longer or until sausage is well done. Remove from pan, drain on paper towels, and add to the sauce mixture.

4. If any sausage grease remains in baking pan, pour it off or use paper towels to soak it up. (Be careful handling that hot pan!)

5. Place olive oil, onions, and mushrooms in pan and stir. Air-fry for 5 minutes or just until tender. Using a slotted spoon, transfer onions and mushrooms from baking pan into the sauce and sausage mixture.

6. Place bell pepper chunks in air fryer oven baking pan and air-fry for 8 minutes or until tender. When done, stir into sauce with sausage and other vegetables.

7. Serve over cooked spaghetti with plenty of Parmesan cheese.

Smokehouse-style Beef Ribs

Servings: 3
Cooking Time: 25 Minutes

Ingredients:

- ¼ teaspoon Mild smoked paprika
- ¼ teaspoon Garlic powder
- ¼ teaspoon Onion powder
- ¼ teaspoon Table salt
- ¼ teaspoon Ground black pepper
- 3 10- to 12-ounce beef back ribs (not beef short ribs)

Directions:

1. Preheat the toaster oven to 350°F .

2. Mix the smoked paprika, garlic powder, onion powder, salt, and pepper in a small bowl until uniform. Massage and pat this mixture onto the ribs.

3. When the machine is at temperature, set the ribs in the air fryer oven in one layer, turning them on their sides if necessary, sort of like they're spooning but with at least ¼ inch air space between them. Air-fry for 25 minutes, turning once, until deep brown and sizzling.

4. Use kitchen tongs to transfer the ribs to a wire rack. Cool for 5 minutes before serving.

Air-fried Roast Beef With Rosemary Roasted Potatoes

Servings: 8
Cooking Time: 60 Minutes

Ingredients:

- 1 (5-pound) top sirloin roast
- salt and freshly ground black pepper
- 1 teaspoon dried thyme
- 2 pounds red potatoes, halved or quartered
- 2 teaspoons olive oil
- 1 teaspoon very finely chopped fresh rosemary, plus more for garnish

Directions:

1. Start by making sure your roast will fit into the air fryer oven without touching the top element. Trim it if you have to in order to get it to fit nicely in your air fryer oven. (You can always save the trimmings for another use, like a beef sandwich.)

2. Preheat the toaster oven to 360°F.

3. Season the beef all over with salt, pepper and thyme. Transfer the seasoned roast to the air fryer oven.

4. Air-fry at 360°F for 20 minutes. Turn the roast over and continue to air-fry at 360°F for another 20 minutes.

5. Toss the potatoes with the olive oil, salt, pepper and fresh rosemary. Turn the roast over again in the air fryer oven and toss the potatoes in around the sides of the roast. Air-fry the roast and potatoes at 360°F for another 20 minutes. Check the internal temperature of the roast with an instant-read thermometer, and continue to roast until the beef is 5° lower than your desired degree of doneness. (Rare – 130°F, Medium – 150°F, Well done – 170°F.) Let the roast rest for 5 to 10 minutes before slicing and serving. While the roast is resting, continue to air-fry the potatoes if desired for extra browning and crispiness.

6. Slice the roast and serve with the potatoes, adding a little more fresh rosemary if desired.

Chipotle-glazed Meat Loaf

Servings: 4
Cooking Time: 65 Minutes

Ingredients:

- 1 ½ pounds lean ground beef
- ¼ cup finely chopped onion
- ½ cup crushed tortilla chips
- 1 teaspoon ground cumin
- ½ teaspoon chili powder
- ½ teaspoon garlic powder
- ½ teaspoon kosher salt
- ¼ teaspoon freshly ground black pepper
- 3 tablespoons chopped pickled jalapeños
- 3 tablespoons chunky salsa
- 1 large egg
- ⅓ cup ketchup
- 3 ½ teaspoons minced chipotle chilies in adobo sauce

Directions:

1. Preheat the toaster oven to 375 °F. Line a 12 x 12-inch baking pan with aluminum foil.

2. Combine the ground beef, onion, tortilla chips, cumin, chili powder, garlic powder, salt, pepper, pickled jalapeños, salsa, and egg in a large bowl, stirring until blended well. Shape the meat mixture into a 9 x 5-inch loaf and place on the prepared pan.

3. Bake, uncovered, for 30 minutes. Carefully remove the meat loaf from the oven and spoon off any collected grease from the pan.

4. Place the ketchup in a small bowl and stir in the chipotle chilies in adobo sauce. Spread the ketchup mixture on top of the meat loaf. Continue to bake for an additional 25 to 35 minutes or until a meat thermometer registers 160 °F. Let stand for 10 minutes before slicing.

Perfect Pork Chops

Servings: 3
Cooking Time: 10 Minutes

Ingredients:

* ¾ teaspoon Mild paprika
* ¾ teaspoon Dried thyme
* ¾ teaspoon Onion powder
* ¼ teaspoon Garlic powder
* ¼ teaspoon Table salt
* ¼ teaspoon Ground black pepper
* 3 6-ounce boneless center-cut pork loin chops
* Vegetable oil spray

Directions:

1. Preheat the toaster oven to 400°F.

2. Mix the paprika, thyme, onion powder, garlic powder, salt, and pepper in a small bowl until well combined. Massage this mixture into both sides of the chops. Generously coat both sides of the chops with vegetable oil spray.

3. When the machine is at temperature, set the chops in the air fryer oven with as much air space between them as possible. Air-fry undisturbed for 10 minutes, or until an instant-read meat thermometer inserted into the thickest part of a chop registers 145°F.

4. Use kitchen tongs to transfer the chops to a cutting board or serving plates. Cool for 5 minutes before serving.

Minted Lamb Chops

Servings: 4
Cooking Time: 15 Minutes

Ingredients:

* Mint mixture:
* 4 tablespoons finely chopped fresh mint
* 2 tablespoons nonfat yogurt
* 1 tablespoon olive oil
* Salt and freshly ground black pepper to taste
* 4 lean lamb chops, fat trimmed, approximately ¾ inch thick
* 1 tablespoon balsamic vinegar

Directions:

1. Combine the mint mixture ingredients in a small bowl, stirring well to blend. Set aside. Place the lamp chops on a broiling rack with a pan underneath.

2. BROIL the lamb chops for 10 minutes, or until they are slightly pink. Remove from the oven and brush one side liberally with balsamic vinegar. Turn the chops over with tongs and spread with the mint mixture, using all of the mixture.

3. BROIL again for 5 minutes, or until lightly browned.

Lamb Koftas Meatballs

Servings: 3
Cooking Time: 8 Minutes

Ingredients:

- 1 pound ground lamb
- 1 teaspoon ground cumin
- 1 teaspoon ground coriander
- 2 tablespoons chopped fresh mint
- 1 egg, beaten
- ½ teaspoon salt
- freshly ground black pepper

Directions:

1. Combine all ingredients in a bowl and mix together well. Divide the mixture into 10 portions. Roll each portion into a ball and then by cupping the meatball in your hand, shape it into an oval.
2. Preheat the toaster oven to 400°F.
3. Air-fry the koftas for 8 minutes.
4. Serve warm with the cucumber-yogurt dip.

Sloppy Joes

Servings: 4
Cooking Time: 17 Minutes

Ingredients:

- oil for misting or cooking spray
- 1 pound very lean ground beef
- 1 teaspoon onion powder
- ⅓ cup ketchup
- ¼ cup water
- ½ teaspoon celery seed
- 1 tablespoon lemon juice
- 1½ teaspoons brown sugar
- 1¼ teaspoons low-sodium Worcestershire sauce
- ½ teaspoon salt (optional)
- ½ teaspoon vinegar
- ⅛ teaspoon dry mustard

- hamburger or slider buns

Directions:

1. Spray air fryer oven with nonstick cooking spray or olive oil.
2. Break raw ground beef into small chunks and pile into air fryer oven.
3. Air-fry at 390°F for 5 minutes. Stir to break apart and cook 3 minutes. Stir and cook 4 minutes longer or until meat is well done.
4. Remove meat from air fryer oven, drain, and use a knife and fork to crumble into small pieces.
5. Give your air fryer oven a quick rinse to remove any bits of meat.
6. Place all the remaining ingredients except the buns in a 6 x 6-inch baking pan and mix together.
7. Add meat and stir well.
8. Air-fry at 330°F for 5 minutes. Stir and air-fry for 2 minutes.
9. Scoop onto buns.

Red Curry Flank Steak

Servings: 4
Cooking Time: 18 Minutes

Ingredients:

- 3 tablespoons red curry paste
- ¼ cup olive oil
- 2 teaspoons grated fresh ginger
- 2 tablespoons soy sauce
- 2 tablespoons rice wine vinegar
- 3 scallions, minced
- 1½ pounds flank steak
- fresh cilantro (or parsley) leaves

Directions:

1. Mix the red curry paste, olive oil, ginger, soy sauce, rice vinegar and scallions together in a bowl. Place the flank steak in a shallow glass dish and pour half the marinade over the steak. Pierce the steak several times with a fork or meat

tenderizer to let the marinade penetrate the meat. Turn the steak over, pour the remaining marinade over the top and pierce the steak several times again. Cover and marinate the steak in the refrigerator for 6 to 8 hours.

2. When you are ready to cook, remove the steak from the refrigerator and let it sit at room temperature for 30 minutes.

3. Preheat the toaster oven to 400°F.

4. Cut the flank steak in half so that it fits more easily into the air fryer oven and transfer both pieces to the air fryer oven. Pour the marinade over the steak. Air-fry for 18 minutes, depending on your preferred degree of doneness of the steak (12 minutes = medium rare). Flip the steak over halfway through the cooking time.

5. When your desired degree of doneness has been reached, remove the steak to a cutting board and let it rest for 5 minutes before slicing. Thinly slice the flank steak against the grain of the meat. Transfer the slices to a serving platter, pour any juice from the bottom of the air fryer oven over the sliced flank steak and sprinkle the fresh cilantro on top.

Extra Crispy Country-style Pork Riblets

Servings: 3
Cooking Time: 30 Minutes

Ingredients:
- ⅓ cup Tapioca flour
- 2½ tablespoons Chile powder
- ¾ teaspoon Table salt (optional)
- 1¼ pounds Boneless country-style pork ribs, cut into 1½-inch chunks
- Vegetable oil spray

Directions:
1. Preheat the toaster oven to 375°F .

2. Mix the tapioca flour, chile powder, and salt (if using) in a large bowl until well combined. Add the country-style rib chunks and toss well to coat thoroughly.

3. When the machine is at temperature, gently shake off any excess tapioca coating from the chunks. Generously coat them on all sides with vegetable oil spray. Arrange the chunks in the air fryer oven in one (admittedly fairly tight) layer. The pieces may touch. Air-fry for 30 minutes, rearranging the pieces at the 10- and 20-minute marks to expose any touching bits, until very crisp and well browned.

4. Gently pour the contents of the pan onto a wire rack. Cool for 5 minutes before serving.

Steak With Herbed Butter

Servings: 2
Cooking Time: 16 Minutes

Ingredients:
- 4 tablespoons unsalted butter, softened
- 1 tablespoon minced flat-leaf (Italian) parsley
- 1 tablespoon chopped fresh chives
- 2 cloves garlic, minced
- 1 teaspoon Worcestershire sauce
- 2 beef strip steaks, cut about 1 ½ inches thick
- 1 tablespoon olive oil
- Kosher salt and freshly ground black pepper

Directions:
1. Combine the butter, parsley, chives, garlic, and Worcestershire sauce in a small bowl until well blended; set aside.

2. Preheat the toaster oven to broil.

3. Brush the steaks with olive oil and season with salt and pepper. Place the steak on the broiler rack set over the broiler pan. Place the pan in the toaster oven, positioning the steaks about 3 to 4 inches below the heating element.

(Depending on your oven and the thickness of the steak, you may need to set the rack to the middle position.) Broil for 6 minutes, turn the steaks over, and broil for an additional 7 minutes. If necessary to reach the desired doneness, turn the steaks over again and broil for an additional 3 minutes or until you reach your desired doneness.

4. Spread the herb butter generously over the steaks. Allow the steaks to stand for 5 to 10 minutes before slicing and serving.

Barbecued Broiled Pork Chops

Servings: 2
Cooking Time: 16 Minutes

Ingredients:
- Barbecue sauce mixture:
- 1 tablespoon ketchup
- ¼ cup dry red wine
- 1 tablespoon vegetable oil
- ⅛ teaspoon smoked flavoring (liquid smoke)
- 1 teaspoon chili powder
- 1 teaspoon ground cumin
- 1 teaspoon brown sugar
- ¼ teaspoon butcher's pepper
- 2 large (6- to 8-ounce) lean pork chops, approximately ¾ to 1 inch thick

Directions:
1. Combine the barbecue sauce mixture ingredients in a small bowl. Brush the chops with the sauce and place on a broiling rack with a pan underneath.

2. BROIL 8 minutes, turn with tongs, and broil for another 8 minutes, or until the meat is cooked to your preference.

Beef Al Carbon (street Taco Meat)

Servings: 6
Cooking Time: 8 Minutes

Ingredients:
- 1½ pounds sirloin steak, cut into ½-inch cubes
- ¾ cup lime juice
- ½ cup extra-virgin olive oil
- 1 teaspoon ground cumin
- 2 teaspoons garlic powder
- 1 teaspoon salt

Directions:
1. In a large bowl, toss together the steak, lime juice, olive oil, cumin, garlic powder, and salt. Allow the meat to marinate for 30 minutes. Drain off all the marinade and pat the meat dry with paper towels.

2. Preheat the toaster oven to 400°F.

3. Place the meat in the air fryer oven and spray with cooking spray. Cook the meat for 5 minutes, toss the meat, and continue cooking another 3 minutes, until slightly crispy.

Indian Fry Bread Tacos

Servings: 4
Cooking Time: 20 Minutes

Ingredients:
- 1 cup all-purpose flour
- 1½ teaspoons salt, divided
- 1½ teaspoons baking powder
- ¼ cup milk
- ¼ cup warm water
- ½ pound lean ground beef
- One 14.5-ounce can pinto beans, drained and rinsed
- 1 tablespoon taco seasoning
- ½ cup shredded cheddar cheese
- 2 cups shredded lettuce
- ¼ cup black olives, chopped
- 1 Roma tomato, diced
- 1 avocado, diced

- 1 lime

Directions:

1. In a large bowl, whisk together the flour, 1 teaspoon of the salt, and baking powder. Make a well in the center and add in the milk and water. Form a ball and gently knead the dough four times. Cover the bowl with a damp towel, and set aside.

2. Preheat the toaster oven to 380°F.

3. In a medium bowl, mix together the ground beef, beans, and taco seasoning. Crumble the meat mixture into the air fryer oven and air-fry for 5 minutes; toss the meat and cook an additional 2 to 3 minutes, or until cooked fully. Place the cooked meat in a bowl for taco assembly; season with the remaining ½ teaspoon salt as desired.

4. On a floured surface, place the dough. Cut the dough into 4 equal parts. Using a rolling pin, roll out each piece of dough to 5 inches in diameter. Spray the dough with cooking spray and place in the air fryer oven, working in batches as needed. Air-fry for 3 minutes, flip over, spray with cooking spray, and air-fry for an additional 1 to 3 minutes, until golden and puffy.

5. To assemble, place the fry breads on a serving platter. Equally divide the meat and bean mixture on top of the fry bread. Divide the cheese, lettuce, olives, tomatoes, and avocado among the four tacos. Squeeze lime over the top prior to serving.

Kielbasa Sausage With Pierogies And Caramelized Onions

Servings: 3
Cooking Time: 30 Minutes

Ingredients:

- 1 Vidalia or sweet onion, sliced
- olive oil
- salt and freshly ground black pepper
- 2 tablespoons butter, cut into small cubes
- 1 teaspoon sugar
- 1 pound light Polish kielbasa sausage, cut into 2-inch chunks
- 1 (13-ounce) package frozen mini pierogies
- 2 teaspoons vegetable or olive oil
- chopped scallions

Directions:

1. Preheat the toaster oven to 400°F.

2. Toss the sliced onions with a little olive oil, salt and pepper and transfer them to the air fryer oven. Dot the onions with pieces of butter and air-fry at 400°F for 2 minutes. Then sprinkle the sugar over the onions and stir. Pour any melted butter from the bottom of the air fryer oven over the onions (do this over the sink – some of the butter will spill through the pan). Continue to air-fry for another 13 minutes, stirring the pan every few minutes to cook the onions evenly.

3. Add the kielbasa chunks to the onions and toss. Air-fry for another 5 minutes. Transfer the kielbasa and onions to a bowl and cover with aluminum foil to keep warm.

4. Toss the frozen pierogies with the vegetable or olive oil and transfer them to the air fryer oven. Air-fry at 400°F for 8 minutes.

5. When the pierogies have finished cooking, return the kielbasa and onions to the air fryer oven and gently toss with the pierogies. Air-fry for 2 more minutes and then transfer everything to a serving platter. Garnish with the chopped scallions and serve hot with the spicy sour cream sauce below.

6. Kielbasa Sausage with Pierogies and Caramelized Onions

Barbecue-style London Broil

Servings: 5

Cooking Time: 17 Minutes

Ingredients:

- ¾ teaspoon Mild smoked paprika
- ¾ teaspoon Dried oregano
- ¾ teaspoon Table salt
- ¾ teaspoon Ground black pepper
- ¼ teaspoon Garlic powder
- ¼ teaspoon Onion powder
- 1½ pounds Beef London broil (in one piece)
- Olive oil spray

Directions:

1. Preheat the toaster oven to 400°F.

2. Mix the smoked paprika, oregano, salt, pepper, garlic powder, and onion powder in a small bowl until uniform.

3. Pat and rub this mixture across all surfaces of the beef. Lightly coat the beef on all sides with olive oil spray.

4. When the machine is at temperature, lay the London broil flat in the air fryer oven and air-fry undisturbed for 8 minutes for the small batch, 10 minutes for the medium batch, or 12 minutes for the large batch for medium-rare, until an instant-read meat thermometer inserted into the center of the meat registers 130°F (not USDA-approved). Add 1, 2, or 3 minutes, respectively (based on the size of the cut) for medium, until an instant-read meat thermometer registers 135°F (not USDA-approved). Or add 3, 4, or 5 minutes respectively for medium, until an instant-read meat thermometer registers 145°F (USDA-approved).

5. Use kitchen tongs to transfer the London broil to a cutting board. Let the meat rest for 10 minutes. It needs a long time for the juices to be reincorporated into the meat's fibers. Carve it against the grain into very thin (less than ¼-inch-thick) slices to serve.

Beer-baked Pork Tenderloin

Servings: 4

Cooking Time: 40 Minutes

Ingredients:

- 1 pound lean pork tenderloin, fat trimmed off
- 3 garlic cloves, minced
- 1 cup good-quality dark ale or beer
- 2 bay leaves
- Salt and freshly cracked black pepper
- Spiced apple slices

Directions:

1. Preheat the toaster oven to 400° F.

2. Place the tenderloin in an 8½ × 8½ × 4-inch ovenproof baking dish. Sprinkle the minced garlic over the pork, pour over the beer, add the bay leaves, and season to taste with the salt and pepper. Cover with aluminum foil.

3. BAKE, covered, for 40 minutes, or until the meat is tender. Discard the bay leaves and serve sliced with the liquid. Garnish with the spiced apple slices.

Steak Pinwheels With Pepper Slaw And Minneapolis Potato Salad

Servings: 4

Cooking Time: 16 Minutes

Ingredients:

- Brushing mixture:
- ½ cup cold strong brewed coffee
- 2 tablespoons molasses
- 1 tablespoon tomato paste
- 2 garlic cloves, minced
- 1 tablespoon olive oil

- Garlic powder
- 1 teaspoon butcher's pepper
- 1 pound lean, boneless beefsteak, flattened to ⅛-inch thickness with a meat mallet or rolling pin (place steak between 2 sheets of heavy-duty plastic wrap)

Directions:

1. Combine the brushing mixture ingredients in a small bowl and set aside.

2. Cut the steak into 2 × 3-inch strips, brush with the mixture, and roll up, securing the edges with toothpicks. Brush again with the mixture and place in an oiled or nonstick 8½ × 8½ × 2-inch square baking (cake) pan.

3. BROIL for 8 minutes, then turn with tongs, brush with the mixture again, and broil for another 8 minutes, or until browned.

Chicken Fried Steak

Servings: 4

Cooking Time: 15 Minutes

Ingredients:

- 2 eggs
- ½ cup buttermilk
- 1½ cups flour
- ¾ teaspoon salt
- ½ teaspoon pepper
- 1 pound beef cube steaks
- salt and pepper
- oil for misting or cooking spray

Directions:

1. Beat together eggs and buttermilk in a shallow dish.

2. In another shallow dish, stir together the flour, ½ teaspoon salt, and ¼ teaspoon pepper.

3. Season cube steaks with remaining salt and pepper to taste. Dip in flour, buttermilk egg wash, and then flour again.

4. Spray both sides of steaks with oil or cooking spray.

5. Cooking in 2 batches, place steaks in air fryer oven in single layer. Air-fry at 360°F for 10 minutes. Spray tops of steaks with oil and cook 5 minutes or until meat is well done.

6. Repeat to cook remaining steaks.

Stuffed Bell Peppers

Servings: 4

Cooking Time: 10 Minutes

Ingredients:

- ¼ pound lean ground pork
- ¾ pound lean ground beef
- ¼ cup onion, minced
- 1 15-ounce can Red Gold crushed tomatoes
- 1 teaspoon Worcestershire sauce
- 1 teaspoon barbeque seasoning
- 1 teaspoon honey
- ½ teaspoon dried basil
- ½ cup cooked brown rice
- ½ teaspoon garlic powder
- ½ teaspoon oregano
- ½ teaspoon salt
- 2 small bell peppers

Directions:

1. Place pork, beef, and onion in air fryer oven baking pan and air-fry at 360°F for 5 minutes.

2. Stir to break apart chunks and cook 3 more minutes. Continue cooking and stirring in 2-minute intervals until meat is well done. Remove from pan and drain.

3. In a small saucepan, combine the tomatoes, Worcestershire, barbeque seasoning, honey, and basil. Stir well to mix in honey and seasonings.

4. In a large bowl, combine the cooked meat mixture, rice, garlic powder, oregano, and salt. Add ¼ cup of the seasoned crushed tomatoes. Stir until well mixed.

5. Cut peppers in half and remove stems and seeds.

6. Stuff each pepper half with one fourth of the meat mixture.

7. Place the peppers in air fryer oven and air-fry for 10 minutes, until peppers are crisp tender.

8. Heat remaining tomato sauce. Serve peppers with warm sauce spooned over top.

POULTRY

Chicken Wellington

Servings: 4
Cooking Time: 30 Minutes

Ingredients:

- 2 small (5- to 6-ounce) boneless, skinless chicken breast halves
- Kosher salt and freshly ground black pepper
- 2 teaspoons Italian seasoning
- 2 tablespoons olive oil
- 3 tablespoons unsalted butter, softened
- 3 ounces cream cheese, softened (about ⅓ cup)
- ¾ cup shredded Monterey Jack cheese
- ¼ cup grated Parmesan cheese
- 1 cup frozen (loose-pack) chopped spinach, thawed and squeezed dry
- ¾ cup chopped canned artichoke hearts, drained
- ½ teaspoon garlic powder
- 1 sheet frozen puff pastry, about 9 inches square, thawed (½ of a 17.3-ounce package)
- 1 large egg, lightly beaten

Directions:

1. Preheat the toaster oven to 425° F. Line a 12 x 12-inch baking pan with parchment paper.
2. Cut the chicken breasts in half lengthwise. Season each piece with the salt, pepper, and Italian seasoning. Fold the thinner end under the larger piece to make the chicken breasts into a rounded shape. Secure with toothpicks.
3. Heat a large skillet over medium-high heat. Add the olive oil and heat. Add the chicken breasts and brown well, turning to brown evenly. Remove from the skillet and set aside to cool. Remove the toothpicks.
4. Stir the butter, cream cheese, Monterey Jack, and Parmesan in a large bowl. Stir in the spinach, artichoke hearts, and garlic powder. Season with salt and pepper.
5. Roll out the puff pastry sheet on a lightly floured board until it makes a 12-inch square. Cut into four equal pieces. Spread one-fourth of the spinach-artichoke mixture on the surface of each pastry square to within ½ inch of all four edges. Place the chicken in the center of each. Gently fold the puff pastry up over the chicken and pinch the edges to seal tightly.
6. Place each chicken bundle, seam side down, on the prepared pan. Brush the top of each bundle lightly with the beaten egg. Bake for 25 to 30 minutes, or until the pastry is golden brown and crisp and a meat thermometer inserted into the chicken reaches 165°F.

Rotisserie-style Chicken

Servings: 4
Cooking Time: 75 Minutes

Ingredients:

- 1 (3-pound) whole chicken
- 1 teaspoon sea salt
- 1 teaspoon paprika
- 1 teaspoon dried thyme
- 1 teaspoon dried rosemary
- ¼ teaspoon freshly ground black pepper
- 2 tablespoons olive oil

Directions:

1. Preheat the toaster oven to 375°F on CONVECTION BAKE for 5 minutes.
2. Line the baking tray with foil.
3. Pat the chicken dry with paper towels and season all over with the salt, paprika, thyme,

74

rosemary, and pepper. Place the chicken on the baking tray and drizzle with olive oil.

4. In position 1, bake for 1 hour and 15 minutes, until golden brown and the internal temperature of a thigh reads 165°F.

5. Let the chicken rest for 10 minutes and serve.

Chicken Schnitzel Dogs

Servings: 4
Cooking Time: 10 Minutes

Ingredients:

- ½ cup flour
- ½ teaspoon salt
- 1 teaspoon marjoram
- 1 teaspoon dried parsley flakes
- ½ teaspoon thyme
- 1 egg
- 1 teaspoon lemon juice
- 1 teaspoon water
- 1 cup breadcrumbs
- 4 chicken tenders, pounded thin
- oil for misting or cooking spray
- 4 whole-grain hotdog buns
- 4 slices Gouda cheese
- 1 small Granny Smith apple, thinly sliced
- ½ cup shredded Napa cabbage
- coleslaw dressing

Directions:

1. In a shallow dish, mix together the flour, salt, marjoram, parsley, and thyme.

2. In another shallow dish, beat together egg, lemon juice, and water.

3. Place breadcrumbs in a third shallow dish.

4. Cut each of the flattened chicken tenders in half lengthwise.

5. Dip flattened chicken strips in flour mixture, then egg wash. Let excess egg drip off and roll in breadcrumbs. Spray both sides with oil or cooking spray.

6. Air-fry at 390°F for 5 minutes. Spray with oil, turn over, and spray other side.

7. Air-fry for 3 to 5 minutes more, until well done and crispy brown.

8. To serve, place 2 schnitzel strips on bottom of each hot dog bun. Top with cheese, sliced apple, and cabbage. Drizzle with coleslaw dressing and top with other half of bun.

Chicken In Mango Sauce

Servings: 2
Cooking Time: 40 Minutes

Ingredients:

- 2 skinless and boneless chicken breast halves
- 1 tablespoon capers
- 1 tablespoon raisins
- Mango mixture:
- 1 cup mango pieces
- 1 teaspoon balsamic vinegar
- ½ teaspoon garlic powder
- 1 teaspoon fresh ginger, peeled and minced
- ½ teaspoon soy sauce
- ½ teaspoon curry powder
- 1 tablespoon pimientos, minced
- Salt and pepper to taste

Directions:

1. Preheat the toaster oven to 375° F.

2. Process the mango mixture ingredients in a food processor or blender until smooth. Transfer to an oiled or nonstick 8½ × 8½ × 2-inch square (cake) pan and add the capers, raisins, and pimientos, stirring well to blend. Add the chicken breasts and spoon the mixture over the breasts to coat well.

3. BAKE for 40 minutes. Serve the breasts with the sauce.

Thai Chicken Drumsticks

Servings: 4
Cooking Time: 20 Minutes

Ingredients:

- 2 tablespoons soy sauce
- ¼ cup rice wine vinegar
- 2 tablespoons chili garlic sauce
- 2 tablespoons sesame oil
- 1 teaspoon minced fresh ginger
- 2 teaspoons sugar
- ½ teaspoon ground coriander
- juice of 1 lime
- 8 chicken drumsticks (about 2½ pounds)
- ¼ cup chopped peanuts
- chopped fresh cilantro
- lime wedges

Directions:

1. Combine the soy sauce, rice wine vinegar, chili sauce, sesame oil, ginger, sugar, coriander and lime juice in a large bowl and mix together. Add the chicken drumsticks and marinate for 30 minutes.

2. Preheat the toaster oven to 370°F.

3. Place the chicken in the air fryer oven. It's ok if the ends of the drumsticks overlap a little. Spoon half of the marinade over the chicken, and reserve the other half.

4. Air-fry for 10 minutes. Turn the chicken over and pour the rest of the marinade over the chicken. Air-fry for an additional 10 minutes.

5. Transfer the chicken to a plate to rest and cool to an edible temperature. Pour the marinade from the bottom of the air fryer oven into a small saucepan and bring it to a simmer over medium-high heat. Simmer the liquid for 2 minutes so that it thickens enough to coat the back of a spoon.

6. Transfer the chicken to a serving platter, pour the sauce over the chicken and sprinkle the chopped peanuts on top. Garnish with chopped cilantro and lime wedges.

Chicken Pot Pie

Servings: 4
Cooking Time: 65 Minutes

Ingredients:

- ¼ cup salted butter
- 1 small sweet onion, chopped
- 1 carrot, chopped
- 1 teaspoon minced garlic
- ¼ cup all-purpose flour
- 1 cup low-sodium chicken broth
- ¼ cup heavy (whipping) cream
- 2 cups diced store-bought rotisserie chicken
- 1 cup frozen peas
- Sea salt, for seasoning
- Freshly ground black pepper, for seasoning
- 1 unbaked store-bought pie crust

Directions:

1. Place the rack in position 1 and preheat the toaster oven to 350°F on BAKE for 5 minutes.

2. Melt the butter in a large saucepan over medium-high heat. Sauté the onion, carrot, and garlic until softened, about 12 minutes. Whisk in the flour to form a thick paste and whisk for 1 minute to cook.

3. Add the broth and whisk until thickened, about 2 minutes. Add the heavy cream, whisking to combine. Add the chicken and peas, and season with salt and pepper.

4. Transfer the filling to a 1½-quart casserole dish and top with the pie crust, tucking the edges into the sides of the casserole dish to completely enclose the filling. Cut 4 or 5 slits in the top of the crust.

5. Bake for 50 minutes until the crust is golden brown and the filling is bubbly. Serve.

Crispy Chicken Parmesan

Servings: 4
Cooking Time: 12 Minutes

Ingredients:
- 4 skinless, boneless chicken breasts, pounded thin to ¼-inch thickness
- 1 teaspoon salt, divided
- ½ teaspoon black pepper, divided
- 1 cup flour
- 2 eggs
- 1 cup panko breadcrumbs
- ½ teaspoon dried oregano
- ½ cup grated Parmesan cheese

Directions:
1. Pat the chicken breasts with a paper towel. Season the chicken with ½ teaspoon of the salt and ¼ teaspoon of the pepper.
2. In a medium bowl, place the flour.
3. In a second bowl, whisk the eggs.
4. In a third bowl, place the breadcrumbs, oregano, cheese, and the remaining ½ teaspoon of salt and ¼ teaspoon of pepper.
5. Dredge the chicken in the flour and shake off the excess. Dip the chicken into the eggs and then into the breadcrumbs. Set the chicken on a plate and repeat with the remaining chicken pieces.
6. Preheat the toaster oven to 360°F.
7. Place the chicken in the air fryer oven and spray liberally with cooking spray. Air-fry for 8 minutes, turn the chicken breasts over, and cook another 4 minutes. When golden brown, check for an internal temperature of 165°F.

Pickle Brined Fried Chicken

Servings: 4
Cooking Time: 47 Minutes

Ingredients:

- 4 bone-in, skin-on chicken legs, cut into drumsticks and thighs (about 3½ pounds)
- pickle juice from a 24-ounce jar of kosher dill pickles
- ½ cup flour
- salt and freshly ground black pepper
- 2 eggs
- 1 cup fine breadcrumbs
- 1 teaspoon salt
- 1 teaspoon freshly ground black pepper
- ½ teaspoon ground paprika
- ⅛ teaspoon ground cayenne pepper
- vegetable or canola oil in a spray bottle

Directions:
1. Place the chicken in a shallow dish and pour the pickle juice over the top. Cover and transfer the chicken to the refrigerator to brine in the pickle juice for 3 to 8 hours.
2. When you are ready to cook, remove the chicken from the refrigerator to let it come to room temperature while you set up a dredging station. Place the flour in a shallow dish and season well with salt and freshly ground black pepper. Whisk the eggs in a second shallow dish. In a third shallow dish, combine the breadcrumbs, salt, pepper, paprika and cayenne pepper.
3. Preheat the toaster oven to 370°F.
4. Remove the chicken from the pickle brine and gently dry it with a clean kitchen towel. Dredge each piece of chicken in the flour, then dip it into the egg mixture, and finally press it into the breadcrumb mixture to coat all sides of the chicken. Place the breaded chicken on a plate or baking sheet and spray each piece all over with vegetable oil.
5. Air-fry the chicken in two batches. Place two chicken thighs and two drumsticks into the air fryer oven. Air-fry for 10 minutes. Then, gently

turn the chicken pieces over and air-fry for another 10 minutes. Remove the chicken pieces and let them rest on plate – do not cover. Repeat with the second batch of chicken, air-frying for 20 minutes, turning the chicken over halfway through.

6. Lower the temperature of the air fryer oven to 340°F. Place the first batch of chicken on top of the second batch already in the air fryer oven and air-fry for an additional 7 minutes. Serve warm and enjoy.

Roasted Game Hens With Vegetable Stuffing

Servings: 2
Cooking Time: 50 Minutes

Ingredients:
*   Stuffing:
*   1 cup multigrain bread crumbs
*   2 tablespoons chopped onion
*   1 carrot, shredded
*   1 celery stalk, shredded
*   1 garlic clove, minced
*   2 tablespoons chopped fresh parsley
*   Salt and freshly ground black pepper to taste
*   2 whole game hens (thawed or fresh), giblets removed, rinsed, and patted dry with paper towels

Directions:
1. Preheat the toaster oven to 350° F.
2. Combine the stuffing ingredients in a medium bowl. Stuff the cavities of the game hens and place them in a baking dish.
3. BAKE, covered, for 45 minutes, or until the meat is tender and the juices run clear when the breast is pierced with a fork.
4. BROIL, uncovered, for 8 minutes, or until lightly browned.

Fried Chicken

Servings: 4
Cooking Time: 40 Minutes

Ingredients:
*   12 skin-on chicken drumsticks
*   1 cup buttermilk
*   1½ cups all-purpose flour
*   1 tablespoon smoked paprika
*   ¾ teaspoon celery salt
*   ¾ teaspoon dried mustard
*   ½ teaspoon garlic powder
*   ½ teaspoon freshly ground black pepper
*   ½ teaspoon sea salt
*   ½ teaspoon dried thyme
*   ¼ teaspoon dried oregano
*   4 large eggs
*   Oil spray (hand-pumped)

Directions:
1. Place the chicken and buttermilk in a medium bowl, cover, and refrigerate for at least 1 hour, up to overnight.
2. Preheat the toaster oven to 375°F on AIR FRY for 5 minutes.
3. In a large bowl, stir the flour, paprika, celery salt, mustard, garlic powder, pepper, salt, thyme, and oregano until well mixed.
4. Beat the eggs until frothy in a medium bowl and set them beside the flour.
5. Place the air-fryer basket in the baking tray and generously spray it with the oil.
6. Dredge a chicken drumstick in the flour, then the eggs, and then in the flour again, thickly coating it, and place the drumstick in the basket. Repeat with 5 more drumsticks and spray them all lightly with the oil on all sides.

7. In position 2, air fry for 20 minutes, turning halfway through, until golden brown and crispy with an internal temperature of 165°F.

8. Repeat with the remaining chicken, covering the cooked chicken loosely with foil to keep it warm. Serve.

Orange-glazed Roast Chicken

Servings: 6
Cooking Time: 100 Minutes

Ingredients:
- 1 3-pound whole chicken, rinsed and patted dry with paper towels
- Brushing mixture:
- 2 tablespoons orange juice concentrate
- 1 tablespoon soy sauce
- 1 tablespoon toasted sesame oil
- 1 teaspoon ground ginger
- Salt and freshly ground black pepper to taste

Directions:
1. Preheat the toaster oven to 400° F.
2. Place the chicken, breast side up, in an oiled or nonstick 8½ × 8½ × 2-inch square (cake) pan and brush with the mixture, which has been combined in a small bowl, reserving the remaining mixture. Cover with aluminum foil.
3. BAKE for 1 hour and 20 minutes. Uncover and brush the chicken with remaining mixture.
4. BAKE, uncovered, for 20 minutes, or until the breast is tender when pierced with a fork and golden brown.

Tandoori Chicken Legs

Servings: 2
Cooking Time: 30 Minutes

Ingredients:
- 1 cup plain yogurt
- 2 cloves garlic, minced
- 1 tablespoon grated fresh ginger
- 2 teaspoons paprika
- 2 teaspoons ground coriander
- 1 teaspoon ground turmeric
- 1 teaspoon salt
- ¼ teaspoon ground cayenne pepper
- juice of 1 lime
- 2 bone-in, skin-on chicken legs
- fresh cilantro leaves

Directions:
1. Make the marinade by combining the yogurt, garlic, ginger, spices and lime juice. Make slashes into the chicken legs to help the marinade penetrate the meat. Pour the marinade over the chicken legs, cover and let the chicken marinate for at least an hour or overnight in the refrigerator.
2. Preheat the toaster oven oven to 380°F.
3. Transfer the chicken legs from the marinade to the air fryer oven, reserving any extra marinade. Air-fry for 15 minutes. Flip the chicken over and pour the remaining marinade over the top. Air-fry for another 15 minutes, watching to make sure it doesn't brown too much. If it does start to get too brown, you can loosely tent the chicken with aluminum foil, tucking the ends of the foil under the chicken to stop it from blowing around.
4. Serve over rice with some fresh cilantro on top.

Marinated Green Pepper And Pineapple Chicken

Servings: 4
Cooking Time: 20 Minutes

Ingredients:
- Marinade:
- 1 teaspoon finely chopped fresh ginger
- 2 garlic cloves, finely chopped
- 1 teaspoon toasted sesame oil

- 1 tablespoon brown sugar
- 2 tablespoons soy sauce
- ¾ cup dry white wine
- 2 skinless, boneless chicken breasts, cut into 1 × 3-inch strips
- 2 tablespoons chopped onion
- 1 bell pepper, chopped
- 1 5-ounce can pineapple chunks, drained
- 2 tablespoons grated unsweetened coconut

Directions:

1. Combine the marinade ingredients in a medium bowl and blend well. Add the chicken strips and spoon the mixture over them. Marinate in the refrigerator for at least 1 hour. Remove the strips from the marinade and place in an oiled or nonstick 8½ × 8½ × 2-inch square (cake) pan. Add the onion and pepper and mix well.

2. BROIL for 8 minutes. Then remove from the oven and, using tongs, turn the chicken, pepper, and onion pieces. (Spoon the reserved marinade over the pieces, if desired.)

3. BROIL again for 8 minutes, or until the chicken, pepper, and onion are cooked through and tender. Add the pineapple chunks and coconut and toss to mix well.

4. BROIL for another 4 minutes, or until the coconut is lightly browned.

Southwest Gluten-free Turkey Meatloaf

Servings: 8
Cooking Time: 35 Minutes

Ingredients:

- 1 pound lean ground turkey
- ¼ cup corn grits
- ¼ cup diced onion
- 1 teaspoon minced garlic
- ½ teaspoon black pepper
- ½ teaspoon salt
- 1 large egg
- ½ cup ketchup
- 4 teaspoons chipotle hot sauce
- ⅓ cup shredded cheddar cheese

Directions:

1. Preheat the toaster oven to 350°F.

2. In a large bowl, mix together the ground turkey, corn grits, onion, garlic, black pepper, and salt.

3. In a small bowl, whisk the egg. Add the egg to the turkey mixture and combine.

4. In a small bowl, mix the ketchup and hot sauce. Set aside.

5. Liberally spray a 9-x-4-inch loaf pan with olive oil spray. Depending on the size of your air fryer oven, you may need to use 2 or 3 mini loaf pans.

6. Spoon the ground turkey mixture into the loaf pan and evenly top with half of the ketchup mixture. Cover with foil and place the meatloaf into the air fryer oven. Air-fry for 30 minutes; remove the foil and discard. Check the internal temperature (it should be nearing 165°F).

7. Coat the top of the meatloaf with the remaining ketchup mixture, and sprinkle the cheese over the top. Place the meatloaf back in the air fryer oven for the remaining 5 minutes (or until the internal temperature reaches 165°F).

8. Remove from the oven and let cool 5 minutes before serving. Serve warm with desired sides.

Hot Thighs

Servings: 4
Cooking Time: 40 Minutes

Ingredients:

- 6 skinless, boneless chicken thighs
- ¼ cup fresh lemon juice

- Seasonings:
- 1 teaspoon garlic powder
- ¼ teaspoon cayenne
- ½ teaspoon chili powder
- 1 teaspoon onion powder
- Salt and freshly ground black pepper to taste

Directions:

1. Preheat the toaster oven to 450° F.
2. Brush the chicken thighs liberally with the lemon juice. Set aside.
3. Combine the seasonings in a small bowl and transfer to a paper or plastic bag. Add the thighs and shake well to coat. Remove from the bag and place in an oiled or nonstick 8½ × 8½ × 2-inch square (cake) pan. Cover the pan with aluminum foil.
4. BAKE, covered, for 20 minutes. Turn the pieces with tongs and bake again for another 20 minutes, or until the meat is tender and lightly browned.

Air-fried Turkey Breast With Cherry Glaze

Servings: 6
Cooking Time: 54 Minutes

Ingredients:

- 1 (5-pound) turkey breast
- 2 teaspoons olive oil
- 1 teaspoon dried thyme
- ½ teaspoon dried sage
- 1 teaspoon salt
- ½ teaspoon freshly ground black pepper
- ½ cup cherry preserves
- 1 tablespoon chopped fresh thyme leaves
- 1 teaspoon soy sauce
- freshly ground black pepper

Directions:

1. All turkeys are built differently, so depending on the turkey breast and how your butcher has prepared it, you may need to trim the bottom of the ribs in order to get the turkey to sit upright in the air fryer oven without touching the heating element. The key to this recipe is getting the right size turkey breast. Once you've managed that, the rest is easy, so make sure your turkey breast fits into the air fryer oven before you Preheat the toaster oven oven.
2. Preheat the toaster oven to 350°F.
3. Brush the turkey breast all over with the olive oil. Combine the thyme, sage, salt and pepper and rub the outside of the turkey breast with the spice mixture.
4. Transfer the seasoned turkey breast to the air fryer oven, breast side up, and air-fry at 350°F for 25 minutes. Turn the turkey breast on its side and air-fry for another 12 minutes. Turn the turkey breast on the opposite side and air-fry for 12 more minutes. The internal temperature of the turkey breast should reach 165°F when fully cooked.
5. While the turkey is air-frying, make the glaze by combining the cherry preserves, fresh thyme, soy sauce and pepper in a small bowl. When the cooking time is up, return the turkey breast to an upright position and brush the glaze all over the turkey. Air-fry for a final 5 minutes, until the skin is nicely browned and crispy. Let the turkey rest, loosely tented with foil, for at least 5 minutes before slicing and serving.

Roast Chicken

Servings: 6
Cooking Time: 90 Minutes

Ingredients:

- Nonstick cooking spray

- 1 whole (3 ½ -pound) chicken
- Grated zest and juice of 1 lemon
- 1 tablespoon olive oil
- 1 ½ teaspoons kosher salt
- 1 teaspoon garlic powder
- ½ teaspoon dried thyme leaves
- ½ teaspoon freshly ground black pepper

Directions:

1. Preheat the toaster oven to 350°F. Spray a 12 x 12-inch baking pan with nonstick cooking spray.

2. Drizzle the chicken cavity with about half of the lemon juice. Place half of the juiced lemon into the chicken cavity. Truss the chicken using kitchen twine.

3. Rub the chicken evenly with the olive oil.

4. Stir the salt, garlic powder, lemon zest, thyme, and pepper in a small bowl. Using your fingertips, rub the seasonings evenly over the chicken. Place the chicken, breast side up, in the prepared pan. Drizzle with the remaining lemon juice.

5. Roast, uncovered, for 1 ¼ hours to 1 ½ hours, or until a meat thermometer registers 165°F. Let stand for 10 minutes before carving.

Fiesta Chicken Plate

Servings: 4
Cooking Time: 15 Minutes

Ingredients:

- 1 pound boneless, skinless chicken breasts (2 large breasts)
- 2 tablespoons lime juice
- 1 teaspoon cumin
- ½ teaspoon salt
- ½ cup grated Pepper Jack cheese
- 1 16-ounce can refried beans
- ½ cup salsa
- 2 cups shredded lettuce
- 1 medium tomato, chopped

- 2 avocados, peeled and sliced
- 1 small onion, sliced into thin rings
- sour cream
- tortilla chips (optional)

Directions:

1. Split each chicken breast in half lengthwise.

2. Mix lime juice, cumin, and salt together and brush on all surfaces of chicken breasts.

3. Place in air fryer oven and air-fry at 390°F for 15 minutes, until well done.

4. Divide the cheese evenly over chicken breasts and air-fry for an additional minute to melt cheese.

5. While chicken is cooking, heat refried beans on stovetop or in microwave.

6. When ready to serve, divide beans among 4 plates. Place chicken breasts on top of beans and spoon salsa over. Arrange the lettuce, tomatoes, and avocados artfully on each plate and scatter with the onion rings.

7. Pass sour cream at the table and serve with tortilla chips if desired.

Light And Lovely Loaf

Servings: 4
Cooking Time: 30 Minutes

Ingredients:

- 2 cups ground chicken or turkey breast
- 1 egg
- ½ cup grated carrot
- ½ cup grated celery
- 1 tablespoon finely chopped onion
- ½ teaspoon garlic powder
- Salt and freshly ground black pepper to taste

Directions:

1. Preheat the toaster oven to 400° F.

2. Blend all ingredients in a bowl, mixing well, and transfer to an oiled or nonstick regular-size 4½ × 8½ × 2¼-inch loaf pan

3. BAKE, uncovered, for 30 minutes, until lightly browned.

Chicken Nuggets

Servings: 20
Cooking Time: 14 Minutes

Ingredients:

- 1 pound boneless, skinless chicken thighs, cut into 1-inch chunks
- ¾ teaspoon salt
- ½ teaspoon black pepper
- ½ teaspoon garlic powder
- ½ teaspoon onion powder
- ½ cup flour
- 2 eggs, beaten
- ½ cup panko breadcrumbs
- 3 tablespoons plain breadcrumbs
- oil for misting or cooking spray

Directions:

1. In the bowl of a food processor, combine chicken, ½ teaspoon salt, pepper, garlic powder, and onion powder. Process in short pulses until chicken is very finely chopped and well blended.

2. Place flour in one shallow dish and beaten eggs in another. In a third dish or plastic bag, mix together the panko crumbs, plain breadcrumbs, and ¼ teaspoon salt.

3. Shape chicken mixture into small nuggets. Dip nuggets in flour, then eggs, then panko crumb mixture.

4. Spray nuggets on both sides with oil or cooking spray and place in air fryer oven in a single layer, close but not overlapping.

5. Air-fry at 360°F for 10 minutes. Spray with oil and cook 4 minutes, until chicken is done and coating is golden brown.

6. Repeat step 5 to cook remaining nuggets.

Sweet-and-sour Chicken

Servings: 6
Cooking Time: 10 Minutes

Ingredients:

- 1 cup pineapple juice
- 1 cup plus 3 tablespoons cornstarch, divided
- ¼ cup sugar
- ¼ cup ketchup
- ¼ cup apple cider vinegar
- 2 tablespoons soy sauce or tamari
- 1 teaspoon garlic powder, divided
- ¼ cup flour
- 1 tablespoon sesame seeds
- ½ teaspoon salt
- ¼ teaspoon ground black pepper
- 2 large eggs
- 2 pounds chicken breasts, cut into 1-inch cubes
- 1 red bell pepper, cut into 1-inch pieces
- 1 carrot, sliced into ¼-inch-thick rounds

Directions:

1. In a medium saucepan, whisk together the pineapple juice, 3 tablespoons of the cornstarch, the sugar, the ketchup, the apple cider vinegar, the soy sauce or tamari, and ½ teaspoon of the garlic powder. Cook over medium-low heat, whisking occasionally as the sauce thickens, about 6 minutes. Stir and set aside while preparing the chicken.

2. Preheat the toaster oven to 370°F.

3. In a medium bowl, place the remaining 1 cup of cornstarch, the flour, the sesame seeds, the salt,

the remaining ½ teaspoon of garlic powder, and the pepper.

4. In a second medium bowl, whisk the eggs.

5. Working in batches, place the cubed chicken in the cornstarch mixture to lightly coat; then dip it into the egg mixture, and return it to the cornstarch mixture. Shake off the excess and place the coated chicken in the air fryer oven. Spray with cooking spray and air-fry for 5 minutes, and spray with more cooking spray. Cook an additional 3 to 5 minutes, or until completely cooked and golden brown.

6. On the last batch of chicken, add the bell pepper and carrot to the air fryer oven and cook with the chicken.

7. Place the cooked chicken and vegetables into a serving bowl and toss with the sweet-and-sour sauce to serve.

Crispy Chicken Tenders

Servings: 4
Cooking Time: 22 Minutes

Ingredients:
- 1 pound boneless, skinless chicken breasts
- ½ cup all-purpose flour
- ½ teaspoon kosher salt
- ¼ teaspoon freshly ground black ground pepper
- 1 large egg, beaten
- 3 tablespoons whole milk
- 1 cup cornflake crumbs
- ½ cup grated Parmesan cheese
- Nonstick cooking spray

Directions:
1. Preheat the toaster oven to 375°F. Line a 12 x 12-inch baking pan with nonstick aluminum foil. (Or if lining the pan with regular foil, spray it with nonstick cooking spray.)

2. Cover the chicken with plastic wrap. Pound the chicken with the flat side of a meat pounder until it is even and about ½ inch thick. Cut the chicken into strips about 1 by 3 inches.

3. Combine the flour, salt, and pepper in a small shallow dish. Place the egg and milk in another small shallow dish and use a fork to combine. Place the cornflake crumbs and Parmesan in a third small shallow dish and combine.

4. Dredge each chicken piece in the flour, then dip in the egg mixture, and then coat with the cornflake crumb mixture. Place the chicken strips in a single layer in the prepared baking pan. Spray the chicken strips generously with nonstick cooking spray.

5. Bake for 10 minutes. Turn the chicken and spray with nonstick cooking spray. Bake for an additional 10 to 12 minutes, or until crisp and a meat thermometer registers 165 °F.

Crispy Curry Chicken Tenders

Servings: 4
Cooking Time: 14 Minutes

Ingredients:
- 1 pound boneless skinless chicken tenders
- ¼ cup plain yogurt
- 2 tablespoons thai red curry paste
- 1½ teaspoons salt, divided
- ½ teaspoon pepper
- 1¾ cups panko breadcrumbs
- 1 teaspoon granulated garlic
- 1 teaspoon granulated onion
- Olive oil or avocado oil spray

Directions:
1. Whisk together the yogurt, curry paste, 1 teaspoon of salt, and pepper in a large bowl. Add the chicken tenders and toss to coat. Cover bowl

with plastic wrap and marinate in the fridge for 6-8 hours.

2. Combine the panko breadcrumbs, ½ teaspoon salt, garlic, and onion. Remove chicken tenders from the marinade and coat individually in the panko mixture.

3. Preheat the toaster oven to 430°F.

4. Spray both sides of each chicken tender well with olive oil or avocado oil spray, then place into the fry basket.

5. Insert the fry basket at mid position in the preheated oven.

6. Select the Air Fry and Shake functions, adjust time to 14 minutes, and press Start/Pause.

7. Flip chicken tenders halfway through cooking. The Shake Reminder will let you know when.

8. Remove when chicken tenders are golden and crispy.

Jerk Chicken Drumsticks

Servings: 2
Cooking Time: 20 Minutes

Ingredients:

- 1 or 2 cloves garlic
- 1 inch of fresh ginger
- 2 serrano peppers, (with seeds if you like it spicy, seeds removed for less heat)
- 1 teaspoon ground allspice
- 1 teaspoon ground nutmeg
- 1 teaspoon chili powder
- ½ teaspoon dried thyme
- ½ teaspoon ground cinnamon
- ½ teaspoon paprika

- 1 tablespoon brown sugar
- 1 teaspoon soy sauce
- 2 tablespoons vegetable oil
- 6 skinless chicken drumsticks

Directions:

1. Combine all the ingredients except the chicken in a small chopper or blender and blend to a paste. Make slashes into the meat of the chicken drumsticks and rub the spice blend all over the chicken (a pair of plastic gloves makes this really easy). Transfer the rubbed chicken to a non-reactive covered container and let the chicken marinate for at least 30 minutes or overnight in the refrigerator.

2. Preheat the toaster oven to 400°F.

3. Transfer the drumsticks to the air fryer oven. Air-fry for 10 minutes. Turn the drumsticks over and air-fry for another 10 minutes. Serve warm with some rice and vegetables or a green salad.

Guiltless Bacon

Servings: 4
Cooking Time: 10 Minutes

Ingredients:

- 6 slices lean turkey bacon, placed on a broiling pan

Directions:

1. BROIL 5 minutes, turn the pieces, and broil again for 5 more minutes, or until done to your preference. Press the slices between paper towels and serve immediately.

VEGETABLES AND VEGETARIAN

Lentil "meat" Loaf

Servings: 4
Cooking Time: 55 Minutes

Ingredients:

- Oil spray (hand-pumped)
- 2 (14-ounce) cans low-sodium lentils, drained and rinsed
- ½ sweet onion, chopped
- 1 carrot, shredded
- 1 teaspoon minced garlic
- 1½ cups seasoned bread crumbs
- ½ cup vegetable broth
- 3 tablespoons tomato paste
- ¼ teaspoon sea salt
- ⅛ teaspoon freshly ground black pepper
- 3 tablespoons ketchup
- 2 tablespoons maple syrup
- 1 tablespoon apple cider vinegar

Directions:

1. Place the rack in position 1 and preheat oven to 375°F on BAKE for 5 minutes.
2. Lightly coat a 9-by-5-inch loaf pan with oil spray.
3. Place the lentils, onion, carrot, and garlic in a food processor and pulse until very well mixed. Transfer the mixture to a large bowl and add the bread crumbs, vegetable broth, tomato paste, salt, and pepper. Mix well. If the mixture doesn't hold together, add vegetable broth by tablespoons until it does.
4. Press the lentil mixture into the loaf pan.
5. In a small bowl, stir the ketchup, maple syrup, and vinegar together. Spread the glaze over the lentil loaf.

6. Bake for 55 minutes until lightly browned. Serve.

Roasted Cauliflower With Garlic And Capers

Servings: 3
Cooking Time: 10 Minutes

Ingredients:

- 3 cups (about 15 ounces) 1-inch cauliflower florets
- 2 tablespoons Olive oil
- 1½ tablespoons Drained and rinsed capers, chopped
- 2 teaspoons Minced garlic
- ¼ teaspoon Table salt
- Up to ¼ teaspoon Red pepper flakes

Directions:

1. Preheat the toaster oven to 375°F .
2. Stir the cauliflower florets, olive oil, capers, garlic, salt, and red pepper flakes in a large bowl until the florets are evenly coated.
3. When the machine is at temperature, put the florets in the pan, spreading them out to as close to one layer as you can. Air-fry for 10 minutes, tossing once to get any covered pieces exposed to the air currents, until tender and lightly browned.
4. Dump the contents of the air fryer oven into a serving bowl or onto a serving platter. Cool for a minute or two before serving.

Steakhouse Baked Potatoes

Servings: 3
Cooking Time: 55 Minutes

Ingredients:

- 3 10-ounce russet potatoes
- 2 tablespoons Olive oil

- 1 teaspoon Table salt

Directions:

1. Preheat the toaster oven to 375°F .

2. Poke holes all over each potato with a fork. Rub the skin of each potato with 2 teaspoons of the olive oil, then sprinkle ¼ teaspoon salt all over each potato.

3. When the machine is at temperature, set the potatoes in the air fryer oven in one layer with as much air space between them as possible. Air-fry for 50 minutes, turning once, or until soft to the touch but with crunchy skins. If the machine is at 360°F, you may need to add up to 5 minutes to the cooking time.

4. Use kitchen tongs to gently transfer the baked potatoes to a wire rack. Cool for 5 or 10 minutes before serving.

Baked Stuffed Potatoes With Vegetables

Servings: 2
Cooking Time: 30 Minutes

Ingredients:

- 2 large baking potatoes, baked, cooled, and pulp scooped out to make shells
- Stuffing:
- 1 carrot, shredded
- ½ bell pepper, seeded and shredded
- 2 tablespoons broccoli, shredded
- 2 tablespoons cauliflower, shredded
- 3 tablespoons fat-free half-and-half
- 1 teaspoon paprika
- ½ teaspoon garlic powder
- ½ teaspoon caraway seeds
- Salt and butcher's pepper to taste

Directions:

1. Preheat the toaster oven to 400° F.

2. Combine the stuffing mixture ingredients, mixing well. Fill the potato shells with the mixture and place the shells in an oiled 8½ × 8½ × 2-inch square baking (cake) pan.

3. BAKE for 25 minutes or until vegetables are cooked.

4. BROIL for 5 minutes, or until the tops are lightly browned.

Simple Roasted Sweet Potatoes

Servings: 2
Cooking Time: 45 Minutes

Ingredients:

- 2 10- to 12-ounce sweet potato(es)

Directions:

1. Preheat the toaster oven to 350°F .

2. Prick the sweet potato(es) in four or five different places with the tines of a flatware fork (not in a line but all around).

3. When the machine is at temperature, set the sweet potato(es) in the air fryer oven with as much air space between them as possible. Air-fry undisturbed for 45 minutes, or until soft when pricked with a fork.

4. Use kitchen tongs to transfer the sweet potato(es) to a wire rack. Cool for 5 minutes before serving.

Hasty Home Fries

Servings: 4
Cooking Time: 20 Minutes

Ingredients:

- 2 medium baking potatoes, scrubbed and finely chopped
- ¼ cup onions, finely chopped
- 1 teaspoon hot sauce
- Salt and freshly ground black pepper

Directions:

1. Combine all the ingredients in a bowl. Transfer the mixture to an oiled or nonstick 8½ × 8½ × 2-inch square baking (cake) pan, adjusting the seasonings to taste.

2. BROIL for 10 minutes, then turn with tongs and broil again for 10 minutes, or until browned and crisped to your preference.

Almond-crusted Spinach Soufflé

Servings: 4
Cooking Time: 25 Minutes

Ingredients:
- 2 tablespoons reduced-fat sour cream
- 1 tablespoon unbleached flour
- 2 cups fresh spinach, rinsed well, drained, and finely chopped, or 1 10-oz. package frozen spinach, thawed, drained, and blotted dry
- 1 egg, separated
- 1 teaspoon olive oil
- Salt and freshly ground black pepper
- Grated nutmeg
- ¼ cup finely chopped almonds

Directions:
1. Preheat the toaster oven to 350° F.

2. Stir together the sour cream and flour in a medium bowl until smooth. Add the spinach, egg yolk, and oil, mixing well and seasoning to taste with the salt, pepper, and nutmeg.

3. Beat the egg white until stiff and fold into the spinach mixture. Pour into a 1-quart 8½ × 8½ × 4-inch ovenproof baking dish. Sprinkle with the almonds.

4. BAKE, uncovered, for 25 minutes, or until firm and the topping is lightly browned.

Roasted Herbed Shiitake Mushrooms

Servings: 5

Cooking Time: 4 Minutes

Ingredients:
- 8 ounces shiitake mushrooms, stems removed and caps roughly chopped
- 1 tablespoon olive oil
- ½ teaspoon salt
- freshly ground black pepper
- 1 teaspoon chopped fresh thyme leaves
- 1 teaspoon chopped fresh oregano
- 1 tablespoon chopped fresh parsley

Directions:
1. Preheat the toaster oven to 400°F.

2. Toss the mushrooms with the olive oil, salt, pepper, thyme and oregano. Air-fry for 5 minutes. The mushrooms will still be somewhat chewy with a meaty texture. If you'd like them a little more tender, add a couple of minutes to this cooking time.

3. Once cooked, add the parsley to the mushrooms and toss. Season again to taste and serve.

Crisp Cajun Potato Wedges

Servings: 2
Cooking Time: 70 Minutes

Ingredients:
- 2 medium baking potatoes, scrubbed, halved, and cut lengthwise into ½-inch-wide wedges
- 1 tablespoon vegetable oil
- Cajun seasonings:
- ¼ teaspoon chili powder
- ⅛ teaspoon cayenne
- ⅛ teaspoon dry mustard
- ⅛ teaspoon salt
- ⅛ teaspoon cumin
- ¼ teaspoon onion powder
- ¼ teaspoon paprika

Directions:

1. Preheat the toaster oven to 450° F.

2. Soak the potato wedges in cold water for 10 minutes to crisp. Drain on paper towels. Brush with the oil.

3. Combine the Cajun seasonings in a small bowl, add the wedges, and toss to coat well. Transfer to an oiled or nonstick 8½ × 8½ × 2-inch square baking (cake) pan.

4. BAKE, covered, for 40 minutes, or until the potatoes are tender. Carefully remove the cover.

5. BROIL for 20 minutes to crisp, turning with a tongs every 5 minutes until the desired crispness is achieved.

Broiled Tomatoes

Servings: 4
Cooking Time: 10 Minutes

Ingredients:
- 2 medium tomatoes
- Filling:
- 2 tablespoons grated Parmesan cheese
- 2 tablespoons bread crumbs
- 2 tablespoons olive oil
- 1 teaspoon dried oregano or 1 tablespoon chopped fresh oregano
- 1 teaspoon garlic powder or 2 garlic cloves, minced
- Salt and freshly ground black pepper to taste

Directions:
1. Slice the tomatoes in half through the stem scar (top) and carefully scoop out the seeds and flesh with a teaspoon. (Remove and discard about 1 tablespoon each.)

2. Mix together the filling ingredients in a small bowl and adjust the seasonings. Fill each tomato half cavity with equal portions of the mixture. Place the tomato halves in an oiled or nonstick 8½ × 8½ × 2-inch square baking (cake) pan.

3. BROIL for 10 minutes, or until the tomatoes are cooked and the tops are browned.

Tasty Golden Potatoes

Servings: 4
Cooking Time: 38 Minutes

Ingredients:
- 2 cups peeled and shredded potatoes
- ½ cup peeled and shredded carrots
- ¼ cup shredded onion
- 1 teaspoon salt
- 1 teaspoon dried rosemary
- 1 teaspoon dried cumin
- 3 tablespoons vegetable oil
- Salt and freshly ground black pepper to taste

Directions:
1. Preheat the toaster oven to 400° F.

2. Mix all the ingredients together in a 1-quart 8½ × 8½ × 2-inch ovenproof baking dish. Adjust the seasonings to taste. Cover the dish with aluminum foil.

3. BAKE, covered, for 30 minutes, or until tender. Remove the cover.

4. BROIL for 8 minutes, or until the top is browned.

Fried Okra

Servings: 4
Cooking Time: 8 Minutes

Ingredients:
- 1 pound okra
- 1 large egg
- 1 tablespoon milk
- 1 teaspoon salt, divided
- ½ teaspoon black pepper, divided
- ¼ teaspoon paprika
- ¼ teaspoon thyme
- ½ cup cornmeal

- ½ cup all-purpose flour

Directions:

1. Preheat the toaster oven to 400°F.

2. Cut the okra into ½-inch rounds.

3. In a medium bowl, whisk together the egg, milk, ½ teaspoon of the salt, and ¼ teaspoon of black pepper. Place the okra into the egg mixture and toss until well coated.

4. In a separate bowl, mix together the remaining ½ teaspoon of salt, the remaining ¼ teaspoon of black pepper, the paprika, the thyme, the cornmeal, and the flour. Working in small batches, dredge the egg-coated okra in the cornmeal mixture until all the okra has been breaded.

5. Place a single layer of okra in the air fryer oven and spray with cooking spray. Air-fry for 4 minutes, toss to check for crispness, and cook another 4 minutes. Repeat in batches, as needed.

Roasted Heirloom Carrots With Orange And Thyme

Servings: 2
Cooking Time: 12 Minutes

Ingredients:

- 10 to 12 heirloom or rainbow carrots (about 1 pound), scrubbed but not peeled
- 1 teaspoon olive oil
- salt and freshly ground black pepper
- 1 tablespoon butter
- 1 teaspoon fresh orange zest
- 1 teaspoon chopped fresh thyme

Directions:

1. Preheat the toaster oven to 400°F.

2. Scrub the carrots and halve them lengthwise. Toss them in the olive oil, season with salt and freshly ground black pepper and transfer to the air fryer oven.

3. Air-fry at 400°F for 12 minutes.

4. As soon as the carrots have finished cooking, add the butter, orange zest and thyme and toss all the ingredients together in the air fryer oven to melt the butter and coat evenly. Serve warm.

Brown Rice And Goat Cheese Croquettes

Servings: 3
Cooking Time: 8 Minutes

Ingredients:

- ¾ cup Water
- 6 tablespoons Raw medium-grain brown rice, such as brown Arborio
- ½ cup Shredded carrot
- ¼ cup Walnut pieces
- 3 tablespoons (about 1½ ounces) Soft goat cheese
- 1 tablespoon Pasteurized egg substitute, such as Egg Beaters (gluten-free, if a concern)
- ¼ teaspoon Dried thyme
- ¼ teaspoon Table salt
- ¼ teaspoon Ground black pepper
- Olive oil spray

Directions:

1. Combine the water, rice, and carrots in a small saucepan set over medium-high heat. Bring to a boil, stirring occasionally. Cover, reduce the heat to very low, and simmer very slowly for 45 minutes, or until the water has been absorbed and the rice is tender. Set aside, covered, for 10 minutes.

2. Scrape the contents of the saucepan into a food processor. Cool for 10 minutes.

3. Preheat the toaster oven to 400°F.

4. Put the nuts, cheese, egg substitute, thyme, salt, and pepper into the food processor. Cover and pulse to a coarse paste, stopping the machine

at least once to scrape down the inside of the canister.

5. Uncover the food processor; scrape down and remove the blade. Using wet, clean hands, form the mixture into two 4-inch-diameter patties for a small batch, three 4-inch-diameter patties for a medium batch, or four 4-inch-diameter patties for a large one. Generously coat both sides of the patties with olive oil spray.

6. Set the patties in the air fryer oven with as much air space between them as possible. Air-fry undisturbed for 8 minutes, or until brown and crisp.

7. Use a nonstick-safe spatula to transfer the croquettes to a wire rack. Cool for 5 minutes before serving.

Cheesy Potato Skins

Servings: 6
Cooking Time: 54 Minutes

Ingredients:

- 3 6- to 8-ounce small russet potatoes
- 3 Thick-cut bacon strips, halved widthwise (gluten-free, if a concern)
- ¾ teaspoon Mild paprika
- ¼ teaspoon Garlic powder
- ¼ teaspoon Table salt
- ¼ teaspoon Ground black pepper
- ½ cup plus 1 tablespoon (a little over 2 ounces) Shredded Cheddar cheese
- 3 tablespoons Thinly sliced trimmed chives
- 6 tablespoons (a little over 1 ounce) Finely grated Parmesan cheese

Directions:

1. Preheat the toaster oven to 375°F .

2. Prick each potato in four places with a fork (not four places in a line but four places all around the potato). Set the potatoes in the air fryer oven with as much air space between them as possible. Air-fry undisturbed for 45 minutes, or until the potatoes are tender when pricked with a fork.

3. Use kitchen tongs to gently transfer the potatoes to a wire rack. Cool for 15 minutes. Maintain the machine's temperature.

4. Lay the bacon strip halves in the air fryer oven in one layer. They may touch but should not overlap. Air-fry undisturbed for 5 minutes, until crisp. Use those same tongs to transfer the bacon pieces to the wire rack. If there's a great deal of rendered bacon fat in the air fryer oven's bottom or on a tray under the pan attachment, pour this into a bowl, cool, and discard. Don't throw it down the drain!

5. Cut the potatoes in half lengthwise (not just slit them open but actually cut in half). Use a flatware spoon to scoop the hot, soft middles into a bowl, leaving ½ inch of potato all around the inside of the spud next to the skin. Sprinkle the inside of the potato "shells" evenly with paprika, garlic powder, salt, and pepper.

6. Chop the bacon pieces into small bits. Sprinkle these along with the Cheddar and chives evenly inside the potato shells. Crumble 2 to 3 tablespoons of the soft potato insides over the filling mixture. Divide the grated Parmesan evenly over the tops of the potatoes.

7. Set the stuffed potatoes in the air fryer oven with as much air space between them as possible. Air-fry undisturbed for 4 minutes, until the cheese melts and lightly browns.

8. Use kitchen tongs to gently transfer the stuffed potato halves to a wire rack. Cool for 5 minutes before serving.

Onions

Servings: 4
Cooking Time: 18 Minutes

Ingredients:

- 2 yellow onions (Vidalia or 1015 recommended)
- salt and pepper
- ¼ teaspoon ground thyme
- ¼ teaspoon smoked paprika
- 2 teaspoons olive oil
- 1 ounce Gruyère cheese, grated

Directions:

1. Peel onions and halve lengthwise (vertically).
2. Sprinkle cut sides of onions with salt, pepper, thyme, and paprika.
3. Place each onion half, cut-surface up, on a large square of aluminum foil. Pull sides of foil up to cup around onion. Drizzle cut surface of onions with oil.
4. Crimp foil at top to seal closed.
5. Place wrapped onions in air fryer oven and air-fry at 390°F for 18 minutes. When done, onions should be soft enough to pierce with fork but still slightly firm.
6. Open foil just enough to sprinkle each onion with grated cheese.
7. Air-fry for 30 seconds to 1 minute to melt cheese.

Buttery Rolls

Servings: 6
Cooking Time: 14 Minutes

Ingredients:

- 6½ tablespoons Room-temperature whole or low-fat milk
- 3 tablespoons plus 1 teaspoon Butter, melted and cooled
- 3 tablespoons plus 1 teaspoon (or 1 medium egg, well beaten) Pasteurized egg substitute, such as Egg Beaters
- 1½ tablespoons Granulated white sugar
- 1¼ teaspoons Instant yeast
- ¼ teaspoon Table salt
- 2 cups, plus more for dusting All-purpose flour
- Vegetable oil
- Additional melted butter, for brushing

Directions:

1. Stir the milk, melted butter, pasteurized egg substitute (or whole egg), sugar, yeast, and salt in a medium bowl to combine. Stir in the flour just until the mixture makes a soft dough.
2. Lightly flour a clean, dry work surface. Turn the dough out onto the work surface. Knead the dough for 5 minutes to develop the gluten.
3. Lightly oil the inside of a clean medium bowl. Gather the dough into a compact ball and set it in the bowl. Turn the dough over so that its surface has oil on it all over. Cover the bowl tightly with plastic wrap and set aside in a warm, draft-free place until the dough has doubled in bulk, about 1½ hours.
4. Punch down the dough, then turn it out onto a clean, dry work surface. Divide it into 5 even balls for a small batch, 6 balls for a medium batch, or 8 balls for a large one.
5. For a small batch, lightly oil the inside of a 6-inch round cake pan and set the balls around its perimeter, separating them as much as possible.
6. For a medium batch, lightly oil the inside of a 7-inch round cake pan and set the balls in it with one ball at its center, separating them as much as possible.
7. For a large batch, lightly oil the inside of an 8-inch round cake pan and set the balls in it with

one at the center, separating them as much as possible.

8. Cover with plastic wrap and set aside to rise for 30 minutes.

9. Preheat the toaster oven to 350°F .

10. Uncover the pan and brush the rolls with a little melted butter, perhaps ½ teaspoon per roll. When the machine is at temperature, set the cake pan in the air fryer oven. Air-fry undisturbed for 14 minutes, or until the rolls have risen and browned.

11. Using kitchen tongs and a nonstick-safe spatula, two hot pads, or silicone baking mitts, transfer the cake pan from the air fryer oven to a wire rack. Cool the rolls in the pan for a minute or two. Turn the rolls out onto a wire rack, set them top side up again, and cool for at least another couple of minutes before serving warm.

Golden Grilled Cheese Tomato Sandwich

Servings: 2
Cooking Time: 10 Minutes

Ingredients:

- 4 slices whole-grain bread
- 4 teaspoons salted butter at room temperature, divided
- 4 to 6 slices cheddar cheese, or your favorite cheese
- 1 large tomato, thinly sliced

Directions:

1. Preheat the toaster oven to 350°F on AIR FRY for 5 minutes.

2. Place the air-fryer basket in the baking sheet and set aside.

3. Butter all four pieces of bread, using 1 teaspoon of butter for each and place 2 pieces of bread, butter-side down, in the basket. Evenly

divide the cheese between the 2 bread slices and top with tomato slices. Place the remaining 2 pieces of bread on the tomatoes, butter-side up.

4. Place the tray in position 2 and air fry for 5 minutes until golden brown. Flip the sandwiches and air fry until the cheese is melted and the other side of the bread is golden brown, about 5 minutes. Serve.

Roasted Belgian Endive With Pistachios And Lemon

Servings: 2
Cooking Time: 7 Minutes

Ingredients:

- 2 Medium 3-ounce Belgian endive head(s)
- 2 tablespoons Olive oil
- ½ teaspoon Table salt
- ¼ cup Finely chopped unsalted shelled pistachios
- Up to 2 teaspoons Lemon juice

Directions:

1. Preheat the toaster oven to 325°F (or 330°F, if that's the closest setting).

2. Trim the Belgian endive head(s), removing the little bit of dried-out stem end but keeping the leaves intact. Quarter the head(s) through the stem (which will hold the leaves intact). Brush the endive quarters with oil, getting it down between the leaves. Sprinkle the quarters with salt.

3. When the machine is at temperature, set the endive quarters cut sides up in the air fryer oven with as much air space between them as possible. They should not touch. Air-fry undisturbed for 7 minutes, or until lightly browned along the edges.

4. Use kitchen tongs to transfer the endive quarters to serving plates or a platter. Sprinkle with the pistachios and lemon juice. Serve warm or at room temperature.

Broccoli With Chinese Mushrooms And Water Chestnuts

Servings: 4

Cooking Time: 20 Minutes

Ingredients:

- 2 cups broccoli florets, cut in half
- ½ cup Chinese dried mushrooms, cooked, drained, stemmed, and sliced
- ¼ cup dry white wine
- 1 5-ounce can sliced water chestnuts, well drained
- 1 tablespoon vegetable oil
- 1 teaspoon toasted sesame oil
- 1 teaspoon oyster sauce

Directions:

1. Combine all the ingredients with ¼ cup water in an oiled or nonstick 8½ × 8½ × 2-inch square baking (cake) pan. Adjust the seasonings to taste.
2. BROIL 20 minutes, turning with tongs every 5 minutes, or until the vegetables are tender.

Roasted Root Vegetables With Cinnamon

Servings: 4

Cooking Time: 20 Minutes

Ingredients:

- 1 small sweet potato, cut into 1-inch pieces
- 2 carrots, cut into 1-inch pieces
- 2 parsnips, cut into 1-inch pieces
- 2 tablespoons brown sugar (dark or light)
- 1 tablespoon olive oil
- ¼ teaspoon ground cinnamon
- Oil spray (hand-pumped)
- Sea salt, for seasoning

Directions:

1. Preheat the toaster oven to 350°F on AIR FRY for 5 minutes.
2. In a large bowl, toss the sweet potato, carrots, parsnips, brown sugar, oil, and cinnamon until well mixed.
3. Place the air-fryer basket in the baking tray and generously spray the mesh with oil.
4. Spread the vegetables in the basket and air fry in position 2 for 20 minutes, shaking the basket after 10 minutes, until the vegetables are tender and lightly caramelized.
5. Season with salt and serve.

Eggplant And Tomato Slices

Servings: 4

Cooking Time: 36 Minutes

Ingredients:

- 2 tablespoons olive oil
- ¼ teaspoon garlic powder
- 4 ½-inch-thick slices eggplant
- 4 ¼-inch-thick slices fresh tomato
- 2 tablespoons tomato sauce or salsa
- ½ cup shredded Parmesan cheese
- Salt and freshly ground black pepper to taste
- 2 tablespoons chopped fresh basil, cilantro, parsley, or oregano

Directions:

1. Whisk together the oil and garlic powder in a small bowl. Brush each eggplant slice with the mixture and place in an oiled or nonstick 8½ × 8½ × 2-inch square baking (cake) pan.
2. BROIL for 20 minutes. Remove the pan from the oven and turn the pieces with tongs. Top each with a slice of tomato and broil another 10 minutes, or until tender. Remove the pan from the oven, brush each slice with tomato sauce or salsa, and sprinkle generously with Parmesan cheese. Season to taste with salt and pepper. Broil again for 6 minutes, until the tops are browned.
3. Garnish with the fresh herb and serve.

Asparagus And Cherry Tomato Quiche

Servings: 4
Cooking Time: 50 Minutes

Ingredients:
- 6 asparagus spears, woody ends removed, cut into 1-inch pieces
- 1 premade unbaked pie crust
- 5 large eggs
- ½ cup half-and-half
- ¾ cup shredded Swiss cheese, divided
- Sea salt, for seasoning
- Freshly ground black pepper, for seasoning
- 10 cherry tomatoes, quartered
- 1 scallion, both white and green parts, finely chopped

Directions:
1. Place the rack in position 1 and preheat oven to 350°F on BAKE for 5 minutes.
2. Place a small saucepan three-quarters filled with water on high heat and bring to a boil. Blanch the asparagus until bright green, about 1 minute. Drain and set aside.
3. Line an 8-inch-round pie dish with the pie crust, then trim and flute the edges.
4. In a small bowl, beat the eggs, half-and-half, and ½ cup of the cheese until well blended; season with salt and pepper.
5. Arrange the asparagus, tomatoes, and scallion in the pie crust. Pour in the egg mixture and top with the remaining ¼ cup of cheese.
6. Bake for 45 to 50 minutes until the quiche is puffed and lightly browned, and a knife inserted in the center comes out clean.
7. Serve warm or cold.

Crispy Brussels Sprouts

Servings: 3
Cooking Time: 12 Minutes

Ingredients:
- 1¼ pounds Medium, 2-inch-in-length Brussels sprouts
- 1½ tablespoons Olive oil
- ¾ teaspoon Table salt

Directions:
1. Preheat the toaster oven to 400°F.
2. Halve each Brussels sprout through the stem end, pulling off and discarding any discolored outer leaves. Put the sprout halves in a large bowl, add the oil and salt, and stir well to coat evenly, until the Brussels sprouts are glistening.
3. When the machine is at temperature, scrape the contents of the bowl into the air fryer oven, gently spreading the Brussels sprout halves into as close to one layer as possible. Air-fry for 12 minutes, gently tossing and rearranging the vegetables twice to get all covered or touching parts exposed to the air currents, until crisp and browned at the edges.
4. Gently pour the contents of the air fryer oven onto a wire rack. Cool for a minute or two before serving.

Salt And Pepper Baked Potatoes

Servings: 40
Cooking Time: 4 Minutes

Ingredients:
- 1 to 2 tablespoons olive oil
- 4 medium russet potatoes (about 9 to 10 ounces each)
- salt and coarsely ground black pepper
- butter, sour cream, chopped fresh chives, scallions or bacon bits (optional)

Directions:

1. Preheat the toaster oven to 400°F.

2. Rub the olive oil all over the potatoes and season them generously with salt and coarsely ground black pepper. Pierce all sides of the potatoes several times with the tines of a fork.

3. Air-fry for 40 minutes, turning the potatoes over halfway through the cooking time.

4. Serve the potatoes, split open with butter, sour cream, fresh chives, scallions or bacon bits.

Roasted Brussels Sprouts With Bacon

Servings: 20

Cooking Time: 4 Minutes

Ingredients:

- 4 slices thick-cut bacon, chopped (about ¼ pound)
- 1 pound Brussels sprouts, halved (or quartered if large)
- freshly ground black pepper

Directions:

1. Preheat the toaster oven to 380°F.

2. Air-fry the bacon for 5 minutes.

3. Add the Brussels sprouts to the air fryer oven and drizzle a little bacon fat from the pan into the air fryer oven. Toss the sprouts to coat with the bacon fat. Air-fry for an additional 15 minutes, or until the Brussels sprouts are tender to a knifepoint.

4. Season with freshly ground black pepper.

DESSERTS

Mixed Berry Hand Pies

Servings: 4
Cooking Time: 15 Minutes

Ingredients:

- ¾ cup sugar
- ½ teaspoon ground cinnamon
- 1 tablespoon cornstarch
- 1 cup blueberries
- 1 cup blackberries
- 1 cup raspberries, divided
- 1 teaspoon water
- 1 package refrigerated pie dough (or your own homemade pie dough)
- 1 egg, beaten

Directions:

1. Combine the sugar, cinnamon, and cornstarch in a small saucepan. Add the blueberries, blackberries, and ½ cup of the raspberries. Toss the berries gently to coat them evenly. Add the teaspoon of water to the saucepan and turn the stovetop on to medium-high heat, stirring occasionally. Once the berries break down, release their juice and start to simmer (about 5 minutes), simmer for another couple of minutes and then transfer the mixture to a bowl, stir in the remaining ½ cup of raspberries and let it cool.

2. Preheat the toaster oven to 370°F.

3. Cut the pie dough into four 5-inch circles and four 6-inch circles.

4. Spread the 6-inch circles on a flat surface. Divide the berry filling between all four circles. Brush the perimeter of the dough circles with a little water. Place the 5-inch circles on top of the filling and press the perimeter of the dough circles together to seal. Roll the edges of the bottom circle up over the top circle to make a crust around the filling. Press a fork around the crust to make decorative indentations and to seal the crust shut. Brush the pies with egg wash and sprinkle a little sugar on top. Poke a small hole in the center of each pie with a paring knife to vent the dough.

5. Air-fry two pies at a time. Brush or spray the air fryer oven with oil and place the pies into the air fryer oven. Air-fry for 9 minutes. Turn the pies over and air-fry for another 6 minutes. Serve warm or at room temperature.

Mississippi Mud Brownies

Servings: 16
Cooking Time: 34 Minutes

Ingredients:

- Nonstick cooking spray
- 3 tablespoons unsweetened cocoa powder
- ¼ cup canola or vegetable oil
- ¼ cup unsalted butter, softened
- 1 cup granulated sugar
- 2 large eggs
- 1 teaspoon pure vanilla extract
- ¾ cup all-purpose flour
- ½ teaspoon table salt
- ½ cup pecan pieces, toasted
- 2 cups mini marshmallows
- FROSTING
- ¼ cup unsalted butter, melted
- 3 tablespoons unsweetened cocoa powder
- ½ teaspoon pure vanilla extract
- 2 cups confectioners' sugar
- 2 to 3 tablespoons whole milk

Directions:

1. Preheat the toaster oven to 350°F. Spray an 8-inch square baking pan with nonstick cooking spray.

2. Beat the cocoa and oil in a large bowl with a handheld mixer at medium speed. Add the butter and mix until smooth. Beat in the granulated sugar. Add the eggs, one at a time, mixing after each addition. Add the vanilla and mix. On low speed, blend in the flour and salt. Stir in the pecans.

3. Pour the batter into the prepared pan. Bake for 28 to 32 minutes, or until a wooden pick inserted into the center comes out clean.

4. Remove the brownies from the oven and sprinkle the marshmallows over the top. Return to the oven and bake for about 2 minutes or until the marshmallows are puffed. Place on a wire rack and let cool completely.

5. Meanwhile, make the frosting: Combine the butter, cocoa, vanilla, confectioners' sugar, and 2 tablespoons milk in a large bowl. Beat until smooth. If needed for the desired consistency, add additional milk. Frost the cooled brownies.

Buttermilk Confetti Cake

Servings: 10-12
Cooking Time: 25 Minutes

Ingredients:
- 1 1/2 cups all purpose flour
- 1/2 teaspoon baking soda
- 1/4 teaspoon salt
- 1/2 cup butter, softened
- 1 cup sugar
- 1 teaspoon vanilla extract
- 2 large eggs
- 3/4 cup buttermilk
- 1/4 cup multi-colored sprinkle
- Cream Cheese Frosting

- Multi-colored sprinkles

Directions:
1. Preheat the toaster oven to 350°F. Grease two 8-inch cake pans and line with parchment paper.

2. Stir flour, baking soda and salt in small bowl. Set mixture aside.

3. Beat butter, sugar and vanilla extract on HIGH in large bowl until blended. Add eggs, one at a time, until well blended.

4. Alternately add flour mixture and buttermilk until combined. Stir in 1/4 cup sprinkles.

5. Divide batter evenly between prepared pans. Place one pan on bottom rack and one pan on top rack, rotate halfway through baking.

6. Bake 20 to 25 minutes or until a toothpick inserted in center of cakes comes out clean. Cool 10 minutes on wire rack.

7. Remove cakes from pans and cool completely on wire racks. Frost with Cream Cheese Frosting and top with sprinkles.

Orange-glazed Brownies

Servings: 12
Cooking Time: 30 Minutes

Ingredients:
- 3 squares unsweetened chocolate
- 3 tablespoons margarine
- 1 cup sugar
- ½ cup orange juice
- 2 eggs
- 1½ cups unbleached flour
- 1 teaspoon baking powder
- Salt to taste
- 1 tablespoon grated orange zest
- Orange Glaze (recipe follows)

Directions:
1. BROIL the chocolate and margarine in an oiled or nonstick 8½ × 8½ × 2-inch square baking

(cake) pan for 3 minutes, or until almost melted. Remove from the oven and stir until completely melted. Transfer the chocolate/margarine mixture to a medium bowl.

2. Beat in the sugar, orange juice, and eggs with an electric mixer. Stir in the flour, baking powder, salt, and orange zest and mix until well blended. Pour into the oiled or nonstick square cake pan.

3. BAKE at 350° F. for 30 minutes, or until a toothpick inserted in the center comes out clean. Make holes over the entire top by piercing with a fork or toothpick. Paint with Orange Glaze and cut into squares.

Orange Strawberry Flan

Servings: 4
Cooking Time: 45 Minutes

Ingredients:
- ¼ cup sugar
- ½ cup concentrated orange juice
- 1 12-ounce can low-fat evaporated milk
- 3 egg yolks
- 1 cup frozen strawberries, thawed and sliced, or 1 cup fresh strawberries, washed, stemmed, and sliced
- 4 fresh mint sprigs

Directions:
1. Preheat the toaster oven to 375° F.

2. Place the sugar in a baking pan and broil for 4 minutes, or until the sugar melts. Remove from the oven, stir briefly, and pour equal portions of the caramelized sugar into four 1-cup-size ovenproof dishes. Set aside.

3. Blend the orange juice, evaporated milk, and egg yolks in a food processor or blender until smooth. Transfer the mixture to a medium bowl and fold in the sliced strawberries. Pour the mixture in equal portions into the four dishes.

4. BAKE for 45 minutes, or until a knife inserted in the center comes out clean. Chill for several hours. The flan may be loosened by running a knife around the edge and inverted on individual plates or served in the dishes. Garnish with fresh mint sprigs.

Heritage Chocolate Chip Cookies

Servings: 16-18
Cooking Time: 12 Minutes

Ingredients:
- 1 1/2 cups all-purpose flour
- 1 teaspoon baking powder
- 1/2 teaspoon salt
- 1 large egg, unbeaten
- 1/2 cup shortening
- 1/2 cup packed dark brown sugar
- 1/4 cup granulated sugar
- 2 teaspoons vanilla extract
- 1 tablespoon milk
- 1 cup chocolate chips

Directions:
1. Preheat the toaster oven to 375ºF.

2. Place all ingredients except chocolate chips in large mixer bowl. With electric mixer on low speed, beat until ingredients are mixed. Gradually increase speed to medium and beat 3 minutes, stopping to scrape bowl as needed.

3. Add chocolate chips and beat on low until blended.

4. Line cookie sheets with parchment paper. Using a small scoop, place 12 scoops of cookie dough about 1-inch apart on parchment.

5. Bake 10 to 12 minutes or until cookies are browned. Slide parchment with baked cookies onto rack to cool. Repeat with remaining dough.

Hasselback Apple Crisp

Servings: 4

Cooking Time: 20 Minutes

Ingredients:

- 2 large Gala apples, peeled, cored and cut in half
- ¼ cup butter, melted
- ½ teaspoon ground cinnamon
- 2 tablespoons sugar
- Topping
- 3 tablespoons butter, melted
- 2 tablespoons brown sugar
- ¼ cup chopped pecans
- 2 tablespoons rolled oats
- 1 tablespoon flour
- vanilla ice cream
- caramel sauce

Directions:

1. Place the apples cut side down on a cutting board. Slicing from stem end to blossom end, make 8 to 10 slits down the apple halves but only slice three quarters of the way through the apple, not all the way through to the cutting board.

2. Preheat the toaster oven to 330°F and pour a little water into the bottom of the air fryer oven drawer. (This will help prevent the grease that drips into the bottom drawer from burning and smoking.)

3. Transfer the apples to the air fryer oven, flat side down. Combine ¼ cup of melted butter, cinnamon and sugar in a small bowl. Brush this butter mixture onto the apples and air-fry at 330°F for 15 minutes. Baste the apples several times with the butter mixture during the cooking process.

4. While the apples are air-frying, make the filling. Combine 3 tablespoons of melted butter with the brown sugar, pecans, rolled oats and flour in a bowl. Stir with a fork until the mixture resembles small crumbles.

5. When the timer on the air fryer oven is up, spoon the topping down the center of the apples. Air-fry at 330°F for an additional 5 minutes.

6. Transfer the apples to a serving plate and serve with vanilla ice cream and caramel sauce.

Honey-roasted Mixed Nuts

Servings: 8

Cooking Time: 15 Minutes

Ingredients:

- ½ cup raw, shelled pistachios
- ½ cup raw almonds
- 1 cup raw walnuts
- 2 tablespoons filtered water
- 2 tablespoons honey
- 1 tablespoon vegetable oil
- 2 tablespoons sugar
- ½ teaspoon salt

Directions:

1. Preheat the toaster oven to 300°F.

2. Lightly spray an air-fryer-safe pan with olive oil; then place the pistachios, almonds, and walnuts inside the pan and place the pan inside the air fryer oven.

3. Air-fry for 15 minutes, every 5 minutes to rotate the nuts.

4. While the nuts are roasting, boil the water in a small pan and stir in the honey and oil. Continue to stir while cooking until the water begins to evaporate and a thick sauce is formed. The sauce should stick to the back of a wooden spoon when mixed. Turn off the heat.

5. Remove the nuts from the air fryer oven (cooking should have just completed) and spoon

the nuts into the stovetop pan. Use a spatula to coat the nuts with the honey syrup.

6. Line a baking sheet with parchment paper and spoon the nuts onto the sheet. Lightly sprinkle the sugar and salt over the nuts and let cool in the refrigerator for at least 2 hours.

7. When the honey and sugar have hardened, store the nuts in an airtight container in the refrigerator.

Blueberry Cheesecake Tartlets

Servings: 9
Cooking Time: 6 Minutes

Ingredients:

- 8 ounces cream cheese, softened
- ¼ cup sugar
- 1 egg
- ½ teaspoon vanilla extract
- zest of 2 lemons, divided
- 9 mini graham cracker tartlet shells
- 2 cups blueberries
- ½ teaspoon ground cinnamon
- juice of ½ lemon
- ¼ cup apricot preserves

Directions:

1. Preheat the toaster oven to 330°F.

2. Combine the cream cheese, sugar, egg, vanilla and the zest of one lemon in a medium bowl and blend until smooth by hand or with an electric hand mixer. Pour the cream cheese mixture into the tartlet shells.

3. Air-fry 3 tartlets at a time at 330°F for 6 minutes, rotating them in the air fryer oven halfway through the cooking time.

4. Combine the blueberries, cinnamon, zest of one lemon and juice of half a lemon in a bowl. Melt the apricot preserves in the microwave or over low heat in a saucepan. Pour the apricot preserves over the blueberries and gently toss to coat.

5. Allow the cheesecakes to cool completely and then top each one with some of the blueberry mixture. Garnish the tartlets with a little sugared lemon peel and refrigerate until you are ready to serve.

Blackberry Pie

Servings: 6
Cooking Time: 30 Minutes

Ingredients:

- Filling:
- 2 16-ounce bags frozen blackberries, thawed, or 2 cups fresh blackberries, washed and well drained
- 1 4-ounce jar baby food prunes
- 2 tablespoons cornstarch
- 3 ¼ cup brown sugar
- 1 tablespoon lemon juice
- Salt to taste
- 1 Graham Cracker Crust, baked (recipe follows)
- Meringue Topping (recipe follows)

Directions:

1. Preheat the toaster oven to 350° F.

2. Combine the filling ingredients in a large bowl, mixing well. Spoon the filling into the baked Graham Cracker Crust and spread evenly.

3. BAKE for 30 minutes. When cool, top with the Meringue Topping.

Strawberry Blueberry Cobbler

Servings: 6
Cooking Time: 30 Minutes

Ingredients:

- Berry filling:

- 1 10-ounce package frozen blueberries, thawed, or 1½ cups fresh blueberries
- 1 10-ounce package frozen strawberries, thawed, or 1½ cups fresh strawberries
- ½ cup strawberry preserves
- ¼ cup unbleached flour
- 1 teaspoon lemon juice
- Topping:
- ¼ cup unbleached flour
- 2 tablespoons margarine
- 1 tablespoon fat-free half-and-half
- ½ teaspoon baking powder
- 1 tablespoon sugar

Directions:

1. Preheat the toaster oven to 400° F.
2. Combine the berry filling ingredients in a large bowl, mixing well. Transfer to an oiled or nonstick 8½ × 8½ × 2-inch square baking (cake) pan. Set aside.
3. Combine the topping ingredients in a small bowl, blending with a fork until the mixture is crumbly. Sprinkle the mixture evenly over the berries.
4. BAKE for 30 minutes, or until the top is lightly browned.

Glazed Apple Crostata

Servings: 6
Cooking Time: 35 Minutes

Ingredients:

- PASTRY
- 1 ¼ cups all-purpose flour
- 3 tablespoons granulated sugar
- ¼ teaspoon table salt
- ½ cup unsalted butter, cut into 1-inch pieces
- 2 ½ to 3 ½ tablespoons ice water
- FILLING
- ¼ cup granulated sugar

- 3 tablespoons all-purpose flour
- ½ teaspoon ground cinnamon
- ¼ teaspoon ground nutmeg
- Dash table salt
- 3 large Granny Smith apples, peeled, cored, and thinly sliced
- 1 tablespoon unsalted butter, cut into small pieces
- 1 large egg
- Coarse white sugar
- GLAZE
- ¼ cup apricot preserves or apple jelly

Directions:

1. Place the flour, sugar, and salt in the work bowl of a food processor. Pulse to combine. Add the butter and pulse until it forms coarse crumbs. With the motor running, drizzle in enough cold water that the mixture comes together and forms a dough. Shape the dough into a disk, wrap in plastic wrap, and refrigerate for at least 1 hour or until chilled.
2. Make the filling: Stir the sugar, flour, cinnamon, nutmeg, and salt in a large bowl. Add the apples and stir to coat; set aside.
3. Preheat the toaster oven to 400°F. Line a 12-inch pizza pan or 12 x 12-inch baking pan with parchment paper.
4. Roll the pastry into a 12-inch circle on a lightly floured board. Gently fold the dough into quarters and transfer to the prepared pan. Unfold the dough. Pile the filling in the center of the pastry, leaving a 1- to 2-inch border around the edges. Dot the apples with the butter. Fold the edges of the crust up around the outer edge of the apples. Whisk the egg in a small bowl, then brush the edges of the crust with the egg. Sprinkle the crust with coarse sugar.

5. Bake for 30 to 35 minutes or until golden brown and the apples are tender.

6. Set on a wire rack. For the glaze, microwave the preserves in a small, microwave-safe glass bowl on High (100 percent) power for 30 seconds or until melted. Pour the preserves through a fine mesh strainer. Brush the warm preserves over the apples (but not over the crust). Serve warm.

Fried Snickers Bars

Servings: 8
Cooking Time: 4 Minutes

Ingredients:

- ⅓ cup All-purpose flour
- 1 Large egg white(s), beaten until foamy
- 1½ cups (6 ounces) Vanilla wafer cookie crumbs
- 8 Fun-size (0.6-ounce/17-gram) Snickers bars, frozen
- Vegetable oil spray

Directions:

1. Preheat the toaster oven to 400°F.

2. Set up and fill three shallow soup plates or small pie plates on your counter: one for the flour, one for the beaten egg white(s), and one for the cookie crumbs.

3. Unwrap the frozen candy bars. Dip one in the flour, turning it to coat on all sides. Gently stir any excess, then set it in the beaten egg white(s). Turn it to coat all sides, even the ends, then let any excess egg white slip back into the rest. Set the candy bar in the cookie crumbs. Turn to coat on all sides, even the ends. Dip the candy bar back in the egg white(s) a second time, then into the cookie crumbs a second time, making sure you have an even coating all around. Coat the covered candy bar all over with vegetable oil spray. Set aside so you can dip and coat the remaining candy bars.

4. Set the coated candy bars in the pan with as much air space between them as possible. Air-fry undisturbed for 4 minutes, or until golden brown.

5. Remove the pan from the machine and let the candy bars cool in the pan for 10 minutes. Use a nonstick-safe spatula to transfer them to a wire rack and cool for 5 minutes more before chowing down.

White Chocolate Cranberry Blondies

Servings: 6
Cooking Time: 18 Minutes

Ingredients:

- ⅓ cup butter
- ½ cup sugar
- 1 teaspoon vanilla extract
- 1 large egg
- 1 cup all-purpose flour
- ½ teaspoon baking powder
- ⅛ teaspoon salt
- ¼ cup dried cranberries
- ¼ cup white chocolate chips

Directions:

1. Preheat the toaster oven to 320°F.

2. In a large bowl, cream the butter with the sugar and vanilla extract. Whisk in the egg and set aside.

3. In a separate bowl, mix the flour with the baking powder and salt. Then gently mix the dry ingredients into the wet. Fold in the cranberries and chocolate chips.

4. Liberally spray an oven-safe 7-inch springform pan with olive oil and pour the batter into the pan.

5. Air-fry for 17 minutes or until a toothpick inserted in the center comes out clean.

6. Remove and let cool 5 minutes before serving.

Campfire Banana Boats

Servings: 4

Cooking Time: 20 Minutes

Ingredients:

- 4 medium, unpeeled ripe bananas
- ¼ cup dark chocolate chips
- 4 teaspoons shredded, unsweetened coconut
- ½ cup mini marshmallows
- 4 graham crackers, chopped

Directions:

1. Preheat the toaster oven to 400°F on BAKE for 5 minutes.
2. Cut the bananas lengthwise through the skin about halfway through. Open the pocket to create a space for the other ingredients.
3. Evenly divide the chocolate, coconut, marshmallows, and graham crackers among the bananas.
4. Tear off four 12-inch squares of foil and place the bananas in the center of each. Crimp the foil around the banana to form a boat.
5. Place the bananas on the baking tray, two at a time, and in position 2, bake for 10 minutes until the fillings are gooey and the banana is warmed through.
6. Repeat with the remaining two bananas and serve.

Blueberry Crisp

Servings: 6

Cooking Time: 13 Minutes

Ingredients:

- 3 cups Fresh or thawed frozen blueberries
- ⅓ cup Granulated white sugar
- 1 tablespoon Instant tapioca
- ⅓ cup All-purpose flour
- ⅓ cup Rolled oats (not quick-cooking or steel-cut)
- ⅓ cup Chopped walnuts or pecans
- ⅓ cup Packed light brown sugar
- 5 tablespoons plus 1 teaspoon (⅔ stick) Butter, melted and cooled
- ¾ teaspoon Ground cinnamon
- ¼ teaspoon Table salt

Directions:

1. Preheat the toaster oven to 400°F.
2. Mix the blueberries, granulated white sugar, and instant tapioca in a 6-inch round cake pan for a small batch, a 7-inch round cake pan for a medium batch, or an 8-inch round cake pan for a large batch.
3. When the machine is at temperature, set the cake pan in the air fryer oven and air-fry undisturbed for 5 minutes, or just until the blueberries begin to bubble.
4. Meanwhile, mix the flour, oats, nuts, brown sugar, butter, cinnamon, and salt in a medium bowl until well combined.
5. When the blueberries have begun to bubble, crumble this flour mixture evenly on top. Continue air-frying undisturbed for 8 minutes, or until the topping has browned a bit and the filling is bubbling.
6. Use two hot pads or silicone baking mitts to transfer the cake pan to a wire rack. Cool for at least 10 minutes or to room temperature before serving.

Chewy Brownies

Servings: 16

Cooking Time: 60 Minutes

Ingredients:

- 3 tablespoons Dutch-processed cocoa powder
- ¾ teaspoon espresso powder (optional)
- ⅓ cup boiling water
- 1 ounce unsweetened chocolate, chopped fine

- 5 tablespoons vegetable oil
- 2 tablespoons unsalted butter, melted and cooled
- 1¼ cups (8¾ ounces) sugar
- 1 large egg plus 1 large yolk
- 1 teaspoon vanilla extract
- ¾ cup (3¾ ounces) plus 2 tablespoons all-purpose flour
- 3 ounces bittersweet chocolate, cut into ½-inch pieces
- ½ teaspoon table salt

Directions:

1. Adjust toaster oven rack to middle position and preheat the toaster oven to 350 degrees. Make foil sling for 8-inch square baking pan by folding 2 long sheets of aluminum foil so each is 8 inches wide. Lay sheets of foil in pan perpendicular to each other, with extra foil hanging over edges of pan. Push foil into corners and up sides of pan, smoothing foil flush to pan. Spray foil with vegetable oil spray.

2. Whisk cocoa; espresso powder, if using; and boiling water together in large bowl until smooth. Add unsweetened chocolate and whisk until chocolate is melted. Whisk in oil and melted butter. (Mixture may look curdled.) Whisk in sugar, egg and yolk, and vanilla until smooth. Add flour, bittersweet chocolate, and salt and mix with rubber spatula until no dry flour remains.

3. Scrape batter into prepared pan, smooth top, and bake until toothpick inserted in center comes out with few moist crumbs attached, 25 to 30 minutes, rotating dish halfway through baking. Transfer pan to wire rack and cool for 1½ hours.

4. Using foil overhang, lift brownies from pan. Return brownies to wire rack and let cool completely, about 1 hour. Cut into 2-inch squares and serve.

Vegan Swedish Cinnamon Rolls (kanelbullar)

Servings: 8
Cooking Time: 18 Minutes

Ingredients:

- Dough
- 1 cup unsweetened almond milk, slightly warm (100°-110°F)
- ¼ cup vegan butter, melted
- 2 tablespoon organic sugar
- 1 teaspoon instant dry yeast
- ½ teaspoon kosher salt
- 2¾ cups all-purpose flour, divided
- Filling
- 6 tablespoons vegan butter, room temperature
- 6 tablespoons organic dark brown sugar
- 1 tablespoon ground cinnamon
- Egg Wash
- 2 tablespoons unsweetened almond milk
- 1 teaspoon agave nectar
- Glaze
- 2 tablespoons unsweetened almond milk
- ½ cup powdered sugar
- ¼ teaspoon vanilla extract
- Swedish pearl sugar, for sprinkling

Directions:

1. Whisk together the almond milk, melted butter, and sugar from the dough ingredients in a large mixing bowl.

2. Sprinkle the yeast into the milk mixture and allow it to bloom for 5 minutes.

3. Add kosher salt and 2¼-cups of flour into the milk and yeast mixture, then mix until well combined.

4. Cover the bowl with a towel or plastic wrap and set in a warm place to rise for 1 hour, or until it doubles in size.

5. Uncover and knead ½-cup all purpose flour into the risen dough. Continue kneading until it just loses its stickiness. You may need to add additional flour.

6. Roll the dough out into a large rectangle, about ½-inch thick. Fix the corners to make sure they are sharp and even.

7. Spread the softened vegan butter from the filling ingredients over the dough and sprinkle evenly with brown sugar and cinnamon.

8. Roll up the dough, forming a log, and pinch the seam closed. Place seam-side down. Trim off any unevenness on either end.

9. Cut the log in half, then divide each half into 8 evenly sized pieces, about 1½-inches thick each.

10. Line the food tray with parchment paper, then place the cinnamon rolls on the tray.

11. Cover with plastic wrap and place in a warm place to rise for 30 minutes.

12. Preheat the toaster Oven to 375°F.

13. Whisk together egg wash ingredients and lightly brush the wash on the tops of the cinnamon rolls.

14. Insert the food tray with the cinnamon rolls at mid position in the preheated oven.

15. Select the Bake function, adjust time to 18 minutes, and press Start/Pause.

16. Remove when done.

17. Whisk together almond milk, powdered sugar, and vanilla extract from the glaze ingredients to make the icing, brush it all over the cinnamon rolls, then sprinkle the rolls with Swedish pearl sugar.

18. Cool before serving, or eat warm.

Pineapple Tartlets

Servings: 4

Cooking Time: 20 Minutes

Ingredients:
- Vegetable oil
- 6 sheets phyllo pastry
- 1 8-ounce can crushed pineapple, drained
- 3 tablespoons low-fat cottage cheese
- 2 tablespoons orange or pineapple marmalade
- 6 teaspoons concentrated thawed frozen orange juice
- Vanilla frozen yogurt or nonfat whipped topping

Directions:
1. Preheat the toaster oven to 350° F.

2. Brush the pans of a 6-muffin tin with vegetable oil. Lay a phyllo sheet on a clean, flat surface and brush with oil. Fold the sheet into quarters to fit the muffin pan. Repeat the process for the remaining phyllo sheets and pans.

3. BAKE for 5 minutes, or until lightly browned. Remove from the oven and cool.

4. Combine the pineapple, cottage cheese, and marmalade in a small bowl, mixing well. Fill the phyllo shells (in the pans) with equal portions of the mixture. Drizzle 1 teaspoon orange juice concentrate over each.

5. BAKE at 400° F. for 15 minutes, or until the filling is cooked. Cool and remove the tartlets carefully from the muffin pans to dessert dishes. Top with vanilla frozen yogurt or nonfat whipped topping.

RECIPE INDEX

Crispy Brussels Sprouts 95
Crispy Chicken Parmesan 77
Crispy Chicken Tenders 84
Crispy Curry Chicken Tenders 84
Crispy Sweet-and-sour Cod Fillets 50
Crispy Wontons 47
Crunchy And Buttery Cod With Ritz® Cracker
Crust 53
Crunchy Baked Chicken Tenders 31
Crunchy Fried Pork Loin Chops 63

E
Easy Oven Lasagne 29
Eggplant And Tomato Slices 94
English Muffins 19
Extra Crispy Country-style Pork Riblets 68

F
Family Favorite Pizza 35
Fiesta Chicken Plate 82
Fish Sticks For Kids 54
Fish Tacos With Jalapeño-lime Sauce 50
Fish With Sun-dried Tomato Pesto 55
Flaky Granola 24
Flounder Fillets 51
Fried Chicken 78
Fried Okra 89
Fried Scallops 56
Fried Snickers Bars 103

G
Gardener's Rice 28
Garlic Basil Bread 18
Garlic Breadsticks 44
Garlic Parmesan Kale Chips 42
Garlic-lemon Shrimp Skewers 52
Glazed Apple Crostata 102

Glazed Pork Tenderloin With Carrots Sheet Pan
Supper 26
Golden Grilled Cheese Tomato Sandwich 93
Granola Three Ways 45
Green Bean Soup 32
Grilled Dagwood 17
Guiltless Bacon 85

H
Harvest Chicken And Rice Casserole 30
Hasselback Apple Crisp 100
Hasty Home Fries 87
Heritage Chocolate Chip Cookies 99
Homemade Beef Enchiladas 26
Honey Bourbon–glazed Pork Chops With Sweet
Potatoes + Apples 36
Honey-roasted Mixed Nuts 100
Horseradish Crusted Salmon 58
Horseradish-crusted Salmon Fillets 56
Hot Italian-style Sub 17
Hot Thighs 80

I
Indian Fry Bread Tacos 69
Italian Baked Stuffed Tomatoes 31
Italian Bread Pizza 27
Italian Meatballs 61
Italian Sausage & Peppers 64

J
Jerk Chicken Drumsticks 85

K
Kasha Loaf 28
Kielbasa Sausage With Pierogies And
Caramelized Onions 70

L
Lamb Koftas Meatballs 67

Lentil "meat" Loaf 86
Light And Lovely Loaf 82
Light Beef Stroganoff 33
Loaded Potato Skins 46

M
Maple Balsamic Glazed Salmon 54
Marinated Catfish 59
Marinated Green Pepper And Pineapple Chicken 79
Minted Lamb Chops 66
Miso-glazed Salmon With Broccoli 34
Mississippi Mud Brownies 97
Mixed Berry Hand Pies 97

N
Narragansett Clam Chowder 29
New York–style Crumb Cake 22
Nutty Whole Wheat Muffins 14

O
One-step Classic Goulash 27
Onions 92
Orange Strawberry Flan 99
Orange-glazed Brownies 98
Orange-glazed Roast Chicken 79
Oven-baked Couscous 36
Oven-poached Salmon 55

P
Parmesan Crusted Tilapia 31
Parmesan Garlic French Fries 44
Perfect Pork Chops 66
Pesto Pizza 32
Pickle Brined Fried Chicken 77
Pineapple Tartlets 106
Popovers 23
Portable Omelet 20
Pretzel-coated Pork Tenderloin 63

Q
Quick Shrimp Scampi 52

R
Red Curry Flank Steak 67
Roast Chicken 81
Roasted Belgian Endive With Pistachios And Lemon 93
Roasted Brussels Sprouts With Bacon 96
Roasted Cauliflower With Garlic And Capers 86
Roasted Game Hens With Vegetable Stuffing 78
Roasted Green Beans With Goat Cheese And Hazelnuts 40
Roasted Heirloom Carrots With Orange And Thyme 90
Roasted Herbed Shiitake Mushrooms 88
Roasted Pumpkin Seeds 46
Roasted Root Vegetables With Cinnamon 94
Rosemary-roasted Potatoes 43
Rotisserie-style Chicken 74

S
Sage, Chicken + Mushroom Pasta Casserole 27
Salt And Pepper Baked Potatoes 95
Savory Sausage Balls 42
Seasoned Boneless Pork Sirloin Chops 63
Sesame Green Beans 39
Sheet Pan Beef Fajitas 33
Sheet Pan Loaded Nachos 35
Sheet-pan Hash Browns 16
Shrimp With Jalapeño Dip 57
Simple Holiday Stuffing 41
Simple Roasted Sweet Potatoes 87
Skirt Steak Fajitas 61
Sloppy Joes 67
Smokehouse-style Beef Ribs 64
Snapper With Capers And Olives 51

Southwest Gluten-free Turkey Meatloaf 80
Spanako Pizza 34
Steak Pinwheels With Pepper Slaw And
Minneapolis Potato Salad 71
Steak With Herbed Butter 68
Steakhouse Baked Potatoes 86
Strawberry Blueberry Cobbler 101
Strawberry Shortcake With Buttermilk Biscuits
15
Stuffed Bell Peppers 72
Stuffed Shrimp 57
Sugar-glazed Walnuts 38
Sweet Chili Shrimp 59
Sweet Potato Casserole 43
Sweet-and-sour Chicken 83
Sweet-hot Pepperoni Pizza 21

T
Tandoori Chicken Legs 79

Tarragon Beef Ragout 34
Tasty Golden Potatoes 89
Thai Chicken Drumsticks 76

V
Vegan Swedish Cinnamon Rolls (kanelbullar)
105
Veggie Cheese Bites 45

W
Warm And Salty Edamame 49
White Chocolate Cranberry Blondies 103
Wild Blueberry Lemon Chia Bread 16

Y
Yeast Dough For Two Pizzas 29

Z
Zucchini Bread 14

Printed in the USA
CPSIA information can be obtained
at www.ICGtesting.com
LVHW081328251123
764905LV00007B/155